CTG
Made
Easy

D0276351

LIVERPOOL
JOHN MOORES UNIVERSITY
AVRIL ROBARTS LRC
TEL. 0151 231 4022

For Churchill Livingstone

Commissioning Editor: Inta Ozols
Project Manager: Ewan Halley
Project Editor: Dinah Thom
Design Direction: Judith Wright

CTG Made Easy

Susan Gauge SRN SCM ONC ADM
Clinical Midwife, Birmingham Women's Healthcare NHS Trust, Birmingham, UK

Christine Henderson MA(Warks) MTD DipN DPHE(Surrey) RM RN
Senior Research Fellow, Women's Health & Midwifery, University of Central England, Birmingham, UK

With a contribution by

Andrew Symon RGN RM MA(Hons) PhD
Clinical Research Fellow, Midwife, Perth Royal Infirmary and University of Dundee, Scotland, UK

Foreword by

Harry Gee MD MRCOG
Senior Lecturer, Department of Fetal Medicine, The University of Birmingham; Honorary Consultant, Birmingham Women's Healthcare NHS Trust, Birmingham, UK

Second Edition

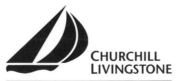

CHURCHILL
LIVINGSTONE

EDINBURGH LONDON NEW YORK PHILADELPHIA SYDNEY TORONTO 1999

CHURCHILL LIVINGSTONE
An imprint of Harcourt Brace and Company Limited

© Harcourt Brace and Company Limited 1999

🖃 is a registered trademark of Harcourt Brace and
Company Limited.

All rights reserved. No part of this publication may be
reproduced, stored in a retrieval system, or transmitted in
any form or by any means, electronic, mechanical,
photocopying, recording or otherwise, without either the
prior permission of the publishers (Harcourt Brace and
Company Limited, 24–28 Oval Road, London NW1 7DX),
or a licence permitting restricted copying in the United
Kingdom issued by the Copyright Licensing Agency, 90
Tottenham Court Road, London W1P 0LP.

First Edition 1992
Second Edition 1999

ISBN 0 443 06148 3

British Library Cataloguing in Publication Data
A catalogue record for this book is available from the
British Library.

Library of Congress Cataloging in Publication Data
A catalog record for this book is available from the Library
of Congress.

Note
Medical knowledge is constantly changing. As new
information becomes available, changes in treatment,
procedures, equipment and the use of drugs become
necessary. The authors and the publishers have, as far as
it is possible, taken care to ensure that the information
given in this text is accurate and up-to-date. However,
readers are strongly advised to confirm that the
information, especially with regard to drug usage, complies
with the latest legislation and standards of practice.

The
publisher's
policy is to use
**paper manufactured
from sustainable forests**

Printed in China

CONTENTS

FOREWORD

In an ideal world we would have a clear understanding of the physiology and pathology of our 'patients'. Our surveillance and testing would be direct, precise and appropriate and we would be able to formulate diagnoses on the basis of this knowledge. Much of medical management, however, is not like this because one, or more, of these aims is not fully achieved, yet the clinical problem remains and treatment has to be given. Under these circumstances the best we can do is make observations and relate them to outcome, i.e. an empirical approach. If there is a reasonable correlation (and there are no set criteria to judge this by) the test would be seen to be of clinical value. However, because a full understanding is lacking, inevitably there will be exceptions which appear to contradict the rules. This does not mean that the test is of little value but, unless the limitations of this approach are acknowledged, the test may be overcriticised despite there being nothing better!

These considerations are applicable to cardiotocography. We are concerned with the ill-effects of hypoxia on the fetus leading to acidosis and, eventually, death. These metabolic changes affect all organ systems of the body but of prime concern is their effect on the brain. The way the fetus responds to adverse changes will depend upon a number of defence mechanisms, e.g. the buffering capacity of body fluids and the ability to rely on anaerobic metabolism. Blood pH value can be determined but usually this is done intermittently and is cumbersome for general surveillance. Oximetry, to measure oxygen saturation of the blood, is under scrutiny but, to date, heart rate monitoring is the most convenient and well-tried method available, albeit an indirect assessment. In *CTG Made Easy* the authors have provided an aid to the more accurate interpretation of heart rate monitoring.

The heart is controlled in a complex way by neurological, endocrine and local mechanisms. The neurological control is mediated by interactions within the brainstem between afferent sensory systems (e.g. baroreceptors, chemoreceptors), higher centres (affected by behavioural states), centres controlling other vital systems (e.g. respiratory activity, thermoregulation) and the efferents via the parasympathetic and sympathetic autonomic nervous systems. It is not the purpose of this Foreword to describe the neurophysiology of heart rate control but only to illustrate the complexity of the interactions which may take place.

Our understanding of these mechanisms has been gleaned from painstaking experimentation, usually using animal models. For these purposes the system under study usually has been isolated from the rest. Even with precise understanding of the response of a single system it can be difficult to predict how the whole organism will respond when all the systems interact with each other. Furthermore, the response may be set by the starting state and this may vary depending on the condition of the fetus. Thus, a growth-retarded fetus with little energy reserve may not behave like its well-nourished counterpart.

Thus, some general rules are known about the fetal response to hypoxia and this knowledge may be employed logically in the interpretation of heart rate recordings. By taking into account factors known to influence heart rate it is possible to improve interpretation. Presumably with better measurement of the physiological status of the fetus, perhaps by monitoring additional important parameters, the proportion of these false predictions could be reduced further but, to date, cardiotocography remains the mainstay of fetal surveillance with the major part of interpretation coming from the rules drawn from empirical correlation of heart rate pattern and fetal condition. As long as this remains the case, any text such as this which aims to improve the accurate interpretation of CTGs should be warmly welcomed.

This second edition has some important additions and the reorganisation of case studies makes *CTG Made Easy* even more relevant.

Birmingham, 1999   Harry Gee

PREFACE

The second edition, whilst following the successful format of the previous edition, has been revised, reorganised and now includes a chapter on 'Litigation and Risk Management'. For those not familiar with the origin of the book the idea of a case study approach to aid the interpretation of cardiotocographs arose in 1986 as a result of the 'Teaching and Assessing in Clinical Practice' course for midwives. A teaching package was produced containing a number of case histories including a section of the cardiotocograph followed by an analysis and description of the management instituted at the time. The package was used extensively in a number of delivery suites by midwives and doctors, initiating lively discussion. We know, from the comments of many doctors and midwives in the UK, that *CTG Made Easy* is used widely, arouses debate and aids learning. The book has an international readership and has been translated into German.

In this second edition we have taken on board the comments of doctors and midwives and have reorganised the text; in particular the case studies have been grouped into categories and some new case studies included. Of great concern within the NHS today is litigation and therefore an important inclusion is a chapter by Andrew Symon on 'Litigation and Risk Management' surrounding CTGs. In line with the underlying philosophy of the book to make it easy for readers, he uses legal cases to illustrate important lessons arising so that we may learn from them. We hope you find the changes helpful and that they will inform your judgements and decision-making in managing care.

Birmingham, 1999   Christine Henderson
Susan Gauge

ACKNOWLEDGEMENT

We would like to thank all those who have helped in the production of this book, especially midwives Annette Gough and Jennifer Henry. We would also like to acknowledge the special contribution of the midwives and doctors on the delivery suite at the Birmingham Women's Healthcare NHS Trust, in particular Judith Weaver, Consultant Obstetrician, and Harold Gee, Clinical Director, for his support.

Introduction to the book

One of the questions uppermost in the minds of mothers, midwives and obstetricians throughout pregnancy and labour is, 'Is the fetus/baby all right?' During labour the fetal heart is either recorded intermittently, using a Pinard's stethoscope, or continuously, using electronic means. This can be external, utilising an external transducer, or internally, with the attachment of a fetal scalp electrode. Monitoring contractions is equally important so that correlation may be made. There is no doubt that the internal means give better contact and produce a more reliable trace. A number of texts already exist which describe fetal physiology and monitoring techniques.

It is not intended in this book to cover in detail the same ground as these texts, but to complement them in initiating discussion by offering a series of examples of traces produced during labour.

This book is for those with some knowledge and experience of fetal heart monitoring during labour and is divided into four parts.

A general overview of CTGs is followed by an interpretation of traces, including a description of abnormalities that could arise.

At the end of Chapter 2 a list of further resources provides the reader with a useful indication of some important sources of information surrounding the issues of fetal well-being. This is followed by a new chapter (Part 2) about 'Litigation and Risk Management' surrounding the cardiotocograph. Legal cases are presented, discussed and important points highlighted. A reference list and extended bibliography are given at the end of the chapter. The third part contains a series of case histories with a portion of the CTG. New case studies have been included. A set of questions to ask concerning the trace are raised for consideration by the reader/group with the opportunity to make notes. An analysis and the management actually instituted at the time is stated. The majority of examples within this book show CTGs with data obtained by means of a fetal scalp electrode and uterine contractions monitored with an intrauterine pressure catheter. We would acknowledge that in current practice these methods are infrequently used. However, for the purpose of interpretation of the CTG, the method by which the data have been obtained in these instances is not important. At the end of the book a summary Risk Assessment Chart is included which summarises the main points for consideration for the practitioner.

The value of the book will be in the richness of the discussions arising from the case studies as presented. This may lead to a review of existing policies and practices. The benefits of such a review will only add to what every mother and baby deserve – practice that is safe, emotionally satisfying and of the highest standard.

PART 1

Understanding the CTG

CHAPTER 1

The cardiotocograph (CTG)

Continuous monitoring of the fetal heart rate during labour became a widespread practice during the 1970s and has remained an accepted technique until relatively recently. Attitudes towards fetal monitoring have altered as more research findings are published highlighting both beneficial and detrimental effects of continuous electronic fetal heart rate monitoring (EFM) (Neilson & Grant 1993, Vintzileos et al 1995). One of the main debates in this arena is the method of EFM used for mothers categorised as low risk or non-complex. It has been shown that for these mothers continuous EFM confers no benefit to the fetus (MacDonald et al 1985), increases operative interventions (Mongelli et al 1997, Supplee & Vezeau 1996, Thacker et al 1995) and with present knowledge its use should be restricted to high-risk or complex cases (Grant 1989).

For low-risk mothers the preferred method of fetal heart rate monitoring is by intermittent auscultation (RCOG 1993), whether this be by the use of a Pinard's stethoscope or hand-held doppler, although the latter may have the benefit of being more comfortable for the mother in allowing her to remain in her chosen position for labour, whilst still allowing the midwife access to estimate the fetal heart rate reliably (Mahomed et al 1994).

Midwives have expressed concern regarding the use of routine continuous EFM during labour (Cooke 1992, Evans 1992). Dover & Gauge (1995) found that, when questioned, midwives stated that intermittent auscultation is their preferred method of fetal monitoring for low-risk mothers in labour; however, when reviewing clinical practice it appears that continuous monitoring by means of abdominal transducers is more widely used. Another study relating to practice and attitudes highlights the ambiguity of the professionals' definition of intermittent fetal monitoring (Birch & Thompson 1997). These findings reiterate an observation made by Murphy-Black (1991) that midwives may have lost their traditional skills in auscultation of the fetal heart. The Royal College of Midwives (RCM) Standing Practice Group (1994) advised midwives to analyse their reasons for using continuous EFM on women in normal labour and to assess procedures in their workplaces. It has been shown that mothers find methods of EFM uncomfortable and restrictive and given a choice would prefer intermittent auscultation as a method of fetal heart rate monitoring (Garcia et al 1985). A mother's choice is important and should be taken into account when discussing and deciding upon the appropriate method of monitoring to be used (DoH 1993, RCOG 1993).

Given the fact that continuous EFM is still used as a method of assessing the well-being of the fetus during labour it is imperative that midwives and medical staff feel confident in correctly interpreting the data on the CTG and instigating the correct management when fetal heart rate abnormalities are detected. A recent confidential enquiry concentrating on intrapartum deaths highlights suboptimal intrapartum care in 75.6% of cases, the most common criticism being the failure to recognise abnormalities occurring on the CTG (CESDI 1997). Another previous study concerned with obstetric litigation also highlighted failure to respond to CTG abnormalities as a problem (Ennis & Vincent 1990). The variability in interpretation between observers is a well-recognised problem when analysing data on the CTG, and suggestions that computerised technology may go some way to eliminating these have been made (Grant 1991).

Having stated that correct interpretation of the data on the CTG is vital to assisting decisions regarding management of labour, it is important that this information is not used in isolation. The progress being made in labour, the amount and colour of any liquor draining and the use of Syntocinon to augment uterine contractions must be taken into account. Failure to observe all of these factors has been noted to be a common problem (Gibb 1997). The Royal College of Obstetricians and Gynaecologists (RCOG 1993) recommend that fetal heart rate monitoring should only be used when facilities are available for fetal blood pH measurements, and ideally estimation of PO_2, PCO_2 and base excess, to allow confirmation of suspected fetal compromise as shown by the CTG. However, this procedure requires skill and can often be uncomfortable for the mother and has the potential for both false positive and negative results (Balen 1993). More recent developments in fetal monitoring methods are being investigated and include the use of pulse oximeters, PCO_2 monitoring and fetal electrocardiography (Cockburn 1996, Groves & Oriol 1995). Until such time as alternative methods have been evaluated EFM remains the foremost method in current use.

The CTG only becomes a valuable method of monitoring and assessment of fetal well-being if the professionals involved are able to interpret the data correctly and have an understanding of the underlying physiology of abnormalities that occur. Regular training in the interpretation of CTG recordings has been advocated for all staff (CESDI 1997, DoH 1994, McDonnell 1997, RCOG 1993), and advice from professional bodies regarding record-keeping and avoidance of litigation claims should be heeded (Chamberlain & Orr 1990, Mason & Edwards 1993).

The interpretation of antenatal and labour CTGs differs. Certain fetal heart rate abnormalities, mainly decelerations, cannot be classified in the absence of uterine contractions, and indeed the physiological explanation for their occurrence may be different. Also during labour the maternal and fetal energy and oxygen requirements change, which places the fetus in a stressful situation. The fetus, in normal circumstances, is able to cope with these changes; however, if a fetus is already compromised before labour begins, the additional stress of uterine contractions diminishes the energy and oxygen flow from the mother to such an extent that fetal compromise occurs. Therefore a fetal heart rate abnormality occurring on an antenatal CTG may require different management from that which would be appropriate if the same abnormality arose during labour. Similarly an abnormality occurring during the early part of labour may warrant different action from that required if the same abnormality arose during the later part of the first stage or second stage. It is also important to view the entire CTG and not just a small portion when analysing the data. Subtle differences such as a slowly rising baseline or gradual decrease in variability may be significant and could be missed. Certain factors can influence the fetal heart rate and affect the management of labour. The following must be considered:

1. Pre-existence of any medical conditions in the mother, e.g.
   Diabetes mellitus
   Renal disease
2. Existence of any pregnancy-related diseases, e.g.
   Pregnancy-induced hypertension
   Rhesus incompatibility

3. Identified risk factors occurring in pregnancy, e.g.
Intrauterine growth retardation
Fetal abnormality
Antepartum haemorrhage
4. Gestational period
5. Progress in labour
6. Any drugs administered to the mother, e.g.
Benzodiazepines (nitrazepam, temazepam)
Tocolytic agents (ritodrine hydrochoride, salbutamol)
Analgesics (pethidine)
7. Posture of the mother throughout the CTG – lying supine will cause a decrease in uterine blood flow, and hence a decrease in oxygen and energy transfer to the fetus.

It is necessary to record certain information on the CTG, to aid in both identification and interpretation:

1. Name and registration number of the mother
2. Date and time of any recording
3. Signature of the doctor or midwife interpreting the CTG
4. Posture of the mother, and changes that occur
5. Speed of the paper, i.e. either 1 cm/min or 3 cm/min
6. All drugs administered to the mother
7. Vaginal examinations, and findings, e.g. cervical dilation, artificial rupture of membranes, state of any liquor observed
8. Blood pressure recordings before and after epidural analgesia
9. Method of monitoring the fetal heart, i.e. internal by means of a fetal scalp electrode, or external by means of an abdominal transducer
10. Method of monitoring uterine activity, i.e. internal by means of an intrauterine pressure catheter, or external by means of an abdominal transducer.

In order to analyse a CTG accurately, the recording must be of good quality. A poor-quality CTG is impossible to interpret; fetal heart rate abnormalities can be missed or mistakenly identified. Uterine activity must be monitored adequately in conjunction with the fetal heart rate. Fetal heart rate abnormalities that occur are classified by relating them to the uterine contractions. If they are not recorded, then an accurate analysis becomes impossible.

If there is any doubt as to the rate of the fetal heart recording on the CTG, it is advisable to auscultate with a Pinard's stethoscope and write the rate on the CTG and check the maternal pulse rate. It is possible for the fetal heart rate monitor to either double count a low fetal heart rate, or to half count a high rate; e.g. a true rate of 60 beats per minute (b.p.m.) may record as 120 b.p.m. or a true rate of 180 b.p.m. may record as 90 b.p.m.

Although unusual, it is possible for the monitor to count the maternal pulse rate. This may occur after the application of a fetal scalp electrode if the fetus is dead (Herbert et al 1987), or with an abdominal transducer even if the fetus is alive.

REFERENCES

Balen A 1993 The value of cardiotocography for intrapartum monitoring. British Journal of Midwifery 1(4): 174–176

Birch L, Thompson B 1997 Survey into fetal monitoring practices and attitudes. British Journal of Midwifery 5(12): 732–736

Chamberlain G, Orr C 1990 How to avoid medico-legal problems in obstetrics and gynaecology. Royal College of Obstetricians and Gynaecologists, London

Cockburn J 1996 The fetal electrocardiogram in the monitoring of fetal well being. Maternal and Child Health 21(1): 14–19

Confidential Enquiry into Stillbirths and Deaths in Infancy (CESDI) 1997 4th annual report. Maternal and Child Health Research Consortium, London

Cooke P 1992 Fetal monitoring – a questionable practice? Modern Midwife 2(2): 8–11

Department of Health (DoH) 1993 Changing childbirth. Report of the Expert Maternity Group. HMSO, London

Department of Health (DoH) 1994 Risk management in the NHS. DoH, London

Dover S L, Gauge S M 1995 Fetal monitoring – midwives' attitudes. Midwifery 11(1): 18–27

Ennis M, Vincent C A 1990 Obstetric accidents: a review of 64 cases. British Medical Journal 300: 1365–1367

Evans S 1992 The value of cardiotocograph monitoring in midwifery. Midwives Chronicle 105(1248): 4–10

Garcia J, Corry M, MacDonald D, Elbourne D, Grant A 1985 Mothers' views on continuous electronic fetal heart rate monitoring and intermittent auscultation in a randomised controlled trial. Birth 21(2): 79–85

Gibb D 1997 Really understanding the cardiotocograph (CTG). Professional Care of Mother and Child 7(5): 125–128

Grant A 1989 Monitoring the fetus during labour. In: Chalmers I, Enkin M, Keirse M (eds) Effective care in pregnancy and childbirth. Oxford University Press, Oxford, pp 846–888

Grant J M 1991 The fetal heart trace is normal, isn't it? Lancet 337: 215–218

Groves P A, Oriol N E 1995 How useful is intrapartum electronic fetal heart rate monitoring. International Journal of Obstetric Anaesthesia 4(3): 161–167

Herbert W N P, Stuart N N, Butler L S 1987 Electronic fetal heart rate monitoring with intrauterine demise. Journal of Obstetric, Gynecologic and Neonatal Nursing 16(4): 249–252

MacDonald D, Grant A, Sheridan-Pereira M, Boylen P, Chalmers I 1985 The Dublin randomised controlled trial of intrapartum fetal heart rate monitoring. American Journal of Obstetrics and Gynecology 52: 524–539

McDonnell R 1997 Risk management in midwifery. MIDIRS Midwifery Digest 7(3): 291–294

Mahomed K, Nyoni R, Mulambo T, Kausle J, Jacobus E 1994 Randomised controlled trial of intrapartum fetal heart rate monitoring. British Medical Journal 308(6927): 497–500

Mason D, Edwards P 1993 Litigation. A risk management guide for midwives. Royal College of Midwives, London

Mongelli M, Chung T K H, Chang A M Z 1997 Obstetric intervention and benefit in conditions of very low prevalence. British Journal of Obstetrics and Gynaecology 104(7): 771–774

Murphy-Black T 1991 Fetal monitoring in labour. Nursing Times 87(28): 58–59

Neilson J P, Grant A M 1993 The randomised trials of intrapartum electronic fetal heart rate monitoring. In: Spencer J A D, Ward R H T (eds) Intrapartum fetal surveillance. RCOG Press, London, pp 77–93

RCM Standing Practice Group 1994 Paper 1: To monitor or not to monitor: the midwife's use of electrocardiographic forms of monitoring the fetus in labour. Midwives Chronicle 107(1276): 189

Royal College of Obstetricians and Gynaecologists 1993 26th RCOG Study Group. Intrapartum fetal surveillance. RCOG Press, London

Supplee R B, Vezeau T M 1996 Continuous electronic fetal monitoring: does it belong in low-risk births? American Journal of Maternal/Child Nursing 21(6): 301–306

Thacker S B, Stroup D F, Peterson H B 1995 Efficacy and safety of intrapartum electronic fetal monitoring: an update. Obstetrics and Gynaecology 86(4): 613–620

Vintzileos A M, Nochimson D J, Guzman E R, Knuppel R A, Lake M, Schifrin B S 1995 Intrapartum electronic fetal heart rate monitoring versus intermittent auscultation: a meta-analysis. Obstetrics and Gynaecology 85(1): 149–154

CHAPTER 2

Interpretation of the CTG

When interpreting a CTG, there are four main points to consider relating to the fetal heart rate:

Basic patterns

1. Baseline heart rate
2. Variability.

Periodic changes

3. Accelerations
4. Decelerations.

In normal circumstances:

1. The baseline heart rate is 110–150 b.p.m.
2. The variability is 5–15 b.p.m.
3. Accelerations may or may not occur in response to uterine contractions or fetal movements
4. No decelerations occur.

Figure 1 shows an example of a normal CTG.

BASIC PATTERNS

Baseline fetal heart rate
This illustrates the rate of the fetal heart, which is controlled mainly by the autonomic nervous system. Sympathetic activity results in tachycardia, while parasympathetic activity, mainly the vagus nerve, results in bradycardia. In normal circumstances, the vagal activity is dominant, exerting a constant slowing of the heart rate, stabilising it at 110–150 b.p.m. The baseline fetal heart is also controlled by receptors in the aortic arch:

1. Chemoreceptors, which are stimulated by changes in oxygen levels. An acute fall in oxygen levels leads to an increase in parasympathetic activity, resulting in a slowing of the heart rate. A more prolonged fall will lead to chronic changes and an increase in sympathetic activity, resulting in a rise in the heart rate.
2. Baroreceptors, which are stimulated by changes in arterial pressure. Hypertension leads to an increase in parasympathetic activity, resulting in a slowing of the heart rate. Hypotension leads to an increase in sympathetic activity, resulting in a rise in the heart rate.

The baseline heart rate is also related to gestational age and the maturity of the vagus nerve. The more mature the fetus, the more evident the slowing effect that the vagus nerve exerts upon the heart rate becomes.

Baseline bradycardia

Definition
Baseline bradycardia is defined as being a persistently low baseline of below 110 b.p.m.

Causes
Many baseline bradycardias have no identifiable cause but there are certain factors that need to be taken into consideration:

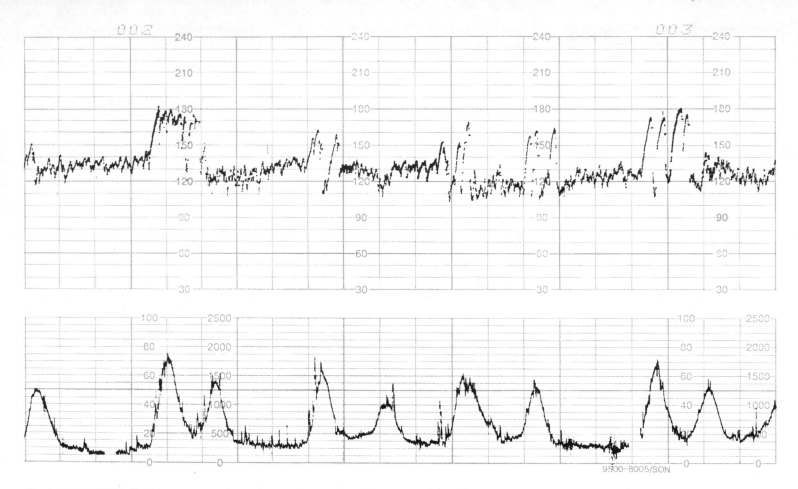

Fig. 1 Normal CTG. Fetal heart recorded using fetal scalp electrode. Contractions recorded using an external transducer. Baseline 125–135 b.p.m.; baseline variability 5–15 b.p.m.; no decelerations, accelerations with some contractions.

1. Gestational age of greater than 40 weeks. Some postmature fetuses have a marked vagal tone, causing a slowing of the heart rate, and can show a baseline bradycardia of 90–110 b.p.m.

2. Cord compression. In cases of acute hypoxia and cord compression a change in the baseline is usually evident from within a normal range to bradycardia.

3. Congenital heart malformations.

4. Certain drugs, e.g. benzodiazepines.

Management
If fetal hypoxia is suspected, a fetal blood sample should be obtained to estimate the pH value and base deficit of the fetal blood. Vaginal examination should be performed to exclude umbilical cord prolapse. Providing that there are no further fetal heart rate abnormalities occurring on the CTG, careful observation is all that is necessary.

Baseline tachycardia

Definition
Baseline tachycardia is defined as being a persistently high baseline of above 150 b.p.m.

Causes
1. *Excessive fetal movements or fetal stimulation.* If the fetus is very active during the period that the CTG is being performed, the fetal heart may not be showing a true baseline. This should be classed as reactivity, but can be mistakenly diagnosed as fetal tachycardia.

2. *Maternal stress and anxiety.* If the mother is in a stressful situation, or has a high anxiety level, she will release catecholamines, thereby stimulating the sympathetic nervous system, resulting in an increase in both maternal and fetal heart rates.

3. *Gestational age.* A fetus at a gestational age of 32 weeks or below can show a baseline tachycardia due to the immaturity of the vagus nerve. The sympathetic nervous system is dominant, resulting in a persistently high fetal heart rate.

4. *Maternal pyrexia.* This is usually associated with maternal tachycardia. Mothers can develop a pyrexia in labour unrelated to infection, particularly if epidural analgesia is used, or if the labour has been long, and signs of maternal distress or obstructed labour are evident. However, with modern management of labour, this should rarely, if ever, be seen. When fetal tachycardia is diagnosed, infection should always be considered.

5. *Fetal infection.* During infection, oxygen requirements are raised. The heart rate rises to increase the oxygen transfer around the body.

6. *Chronic hypoxia.* Chronic changes in the levels of oxygen tension lead to an increase in the sympathetic activity, resulting in a rise in the heart rate. In this instance, the tachycardia may also be complicated by a decrease in variability.

7. *Fetal hormones.* The fetus, in response to stressful situations, e.g. a decrease in oxygen levels, can produce hormones from the adrenal glands, adrenaline and noradrenaline. Their effect is similar to an increase in sympathetic activity, that is, a rise in the heart rate. Therefore, a baseline tachycardia can also be the initial response to fetal hypoxia.

Management

1. Record maternal temperature and pulse rate to exclude pyrexia. If infection is suspected then appropriate treatment should be initiated.

2. If fetal hypoxia is suspected, a fetal blood sample should be obtained to assess the pH value and base excess of the fetal blood, particularly if any other fetal heart rate abnormalities are present. The value of fetal blood sampling in the presence of maternal pyrexia is questionable.

Providing that no further fetal heart rate abnormalities are present, careful observation of the trace is all that is necessary.

Variability

Definition
Variability is due to interaction between all the systems previously described and occurs

as a result of the beat-to-beat changes in the heart rate. Normal variability is between 5–15 b.p.m. (see Fig. 1).

Variability can be measured by analysing a 1-minute portion of a CTG, and assessing the amplitude of change in the heart rate during that period, i.e. the difference in the number of beats per minute of the fetal heart from the highest rate to the lowest rate (any accelerations and decelerations should be excluded; e.g. if the highest rate is 160 b.p.m. and the lowest rate is 155 b.p.m. the difference is 5 b.p.m.).

Aetiology
Variability represents the constant interaction of the sympathetic and parasympathetic nervous systems as they determine the appropriate heart rate and cardiac output in response to constant minor changes in venous return and metabolic demands of the fetus. Normal variability represents an intact nervous pathway through the cerebral cortex, midbrain, vagus nerve and cardiac conduction system. Variability is likely to occur as a result of numerous inputs transmitted through these areas of the nervous system.

Variability can be analysed as being:

1. Normal
2. Increased
3. Decreased.

In order for variability to be interpreted correctly, the heart rate must be monitored on a beat-to-beat basis, by the use of direct fetal electrocardiograph monitoring, achieved by the application of a fetal scalp electrode. When monitoring the fetal heart by means of an abdominal transducer, the monitor recognises each heart beat from a series of echoes and uses the strongest of these to measure the heart rate. The strongest echo may not occur at the same time in every heart beat, resulting in inaccurate measurements of the fetal heart rate variability.

Increased variability

Causes
The initial fetal response to acute hypoxia may cause a transient increase in variability due to stimulation of the parasympathetic nervous system.

Decreased variability

Causes
1. *Fetal sleep.* During fetal sleep the CTG may give an appearance of decreased variability; this should not be confused with lack of reactivity. This pattern should not persist for longer than 30 minutes, after which time the variability should return to within normal limits.

2. *Administration of drugs to the mother.* Decreased variability can be seen following the administration of pethidine to the mother in labour, or of sedative drugs. This pattern

should not persist for longer than 30–40 minutes. Variability should then return to normal.

3. *Gestational age.* The CTG of a fetus at a gestational age of less than 28–30 weeks may show decreased variability, most probably due to the immaturity of the autonomic nervous system.

4. *Severe hypoxia.* When the fetus is suffering from severe or chronic hypoxia the autonomic nervous system fails to respond to stress and the changes in venous return and metabolic demands of the fetus. This is due to a reduction in the transmission of impulses through the nervous system. In the presence of cerebral hypoxia, variability is often severely diminished or absent.

Management
When diminished variability is diagnosed on a CTG, providing any obvious causes, such as administration of pethidine, can be eliminated, fetal hypoxia must always be considered as a cause. Fetal blood sampling should be performed to assess the pH value and base excess of the blood.

The baseline fetal heart rate and variability together are useful indicators of fetal oxygenation. Normal variability represents a fully functioning nervous system. Even in the presence of other fetal heart rate abnormalities suggestive of hypoxia, if the variability is within normal limits, the outcome is usually good.

In the instance of chronic fetal cerebral hypoxia, a decrease or absence of variability may be the only fetal heart rate abnormality present.

Sinusoidal pattern

Sinusoidal patterns may not be viewed as a precise group by some, rather as a subgroup, as there is an increasing tendency today to analyse fetal heart rate according to the frequency of oscillations.

In a study by Young et al (1980) true sinusoidal patterns were uncommon, occurring in only 0.3% of monitored labours. Nonetheless, they do occur and it is important to recognise such a pattern when it occurs.

Definition

This pattern is identifiable by its distinctive smooth, undulating sine-wave-like baseline. Beat-to-beat variability is absent. Figure 2 shows an example CTG exhibiting a sinusoidal pattern.

Aetiology

It is thought that this pattern may be a result of cord compression, resulting in alternating hypervolaemia and hypovolaemia, or of a raised intraperitoneal pressure due to the presence of ascites, resulting in a reduction and eventual cessation of umbilical venous blood flow. In both instances, significant fetal hypoxia will result (O'Connor et al 1980).

Causes

These would fall into three areas: severe hypoxia, anaemia and idiopathic.

Idiopathic. This pattern can be seen as a result of fetal thumb-sucking, and is sometimes seen following the administration of narcotic analgesia to the mother. In these cases the pattern should not persist for longer than 20–30 minutes before a return to normal variability.

Anaemia. The fetus presenting as anaemic, particularly as a result of rhesus incompatibility, twin-to-twin transfusion or large fetomaternal bleed, may produce a sinusoidal pattern.

O'Connor et al (1980) point out, following a review of the literature, that sinusoidal tracings where the oscillations have an amplitude of 20 beats or more, and a frequency of 1–2 oscillations per minute are more suggestive of fetal hypoxia and are an indication for immediate delivery.

Sinusoidal traces where the amplitude of the oscillations is 10 beats or less, with a frequency of 3–5 per minute, may be due to fetal anaemia or thumb-sucking. They can be referred to as pseudosinusoidal and do not usually require immediate action. However, if other fetal heart rate abnormalities are present, delivery should not be delayed.

Management

This pattern should always be regarded as sinister until proven otherwise. A fetal blood sample should be obtained to assess the pH value and base excess of the fetal blood.

If the pattern persists it is an indication for immediate delivery.

PERIODIC CHANGES

Accelerations

Definition

An acceleration is an increase in the fetal heart rate of 15 b.p.m. or more, lasting for at least 15 seconds. Accelerations usually occur in a response to either a fetal movement or a uterine contraction. When accelerations occur the CTG is said to be reactive.

Aetiology

The reaction is caused by the interaction of the sympathetic and parasympathetic nervous systems as a result of an increase in metabolic demands of the fetus during an active phase, or during a uterine contraction in response to compression of the umbilical cord and fetal trunk.

Increased reactivity

This can be due to a period of excessive fetal movements. On analysis of the CTG, increased reactivity can be mistakenly identified as baseline tachycardia.

Decreased reactivity

This can be due to either a period of fetal sleep or the administration of sedation or

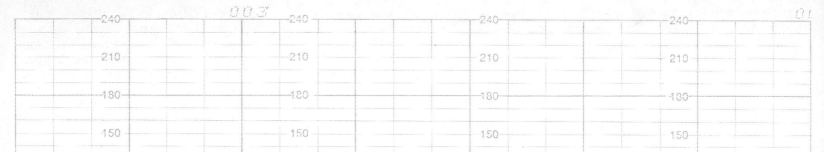
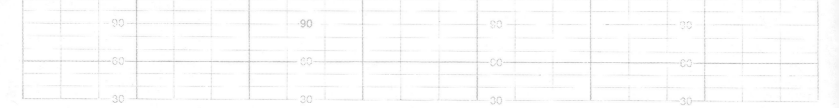
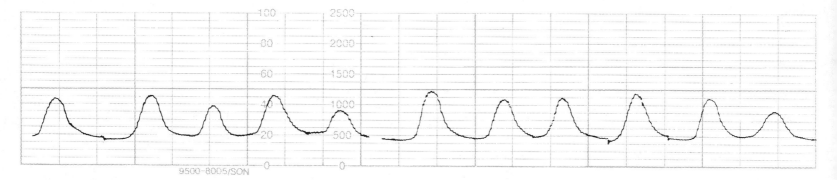

Fig. 2 *Sinusoidal pattern.*

analgesia to the mother. Methods of fetal stimulation, such as abdominal palpation or giving the mother cold water to drink, can evoke a response in the fetus.

It is important not to confuse decreased reactivity with decreased variability. A CTG can be non-reactive but still show variability within normal limits.

Decelerations

Decelerations of the fetal heart rate from the baseline can be classified into four types:

1. Early deceleration
2. Late deceleration
3. Variable deceleration
4. Prolonged deceleration.

The definition and physiological explanation for each type of deceleration is different. It is important to classify them accurately in order for the most effective management to be initiated. Uterine contractions must be monitored adequately in order for the deceleration to be classified.

Early decelerations

Definition. The onset of the deceleration is at the onset of the contraction. The heart rate reaches its lowest point at the peak of the contraction and has recovered to the baseline by the end of the contraction. The amplitude of the deceleration is 40 b.p.m. or less. Figure 3 shows an example CTG exhibiting early decelerations.

Aetiology. Early decelerations are caused by compression of the fetal head during a contraction. Compression of the fetal head causes an increase in intracranial pressure and therefore a decrease in cerebral blood flow and oxygenation. The decrease in oxygen tension is detected by cerebral chemoreceptors, and parasympathetic activity is increased, resulting in a fall in the fetal heart rate. During head compression, pressure on the vagal centre in the brain may also occur, increasing parasympathetic activity.

These decelerations are caused by a mild, transient hypoxia and are not associated with a poor fetal outcome.

Management. This is aimed at relieving the pressure on the fetal head during a uterine contraction. Changing the maternal posture is normally all that is required.

Late decelerations

Definition. Any deceleration whose lowest point occurs more than 15 seconds after the peak of the contraction is said to be late (for an example CTG, see Fig. 4).

Aetiology. Late decelerations arise as a result of a decrease in uterine blood flow and therefore oxygen transfer during a uterine contraction. The low oxygen tension is detected by chemoreceptors in the aortic arch, resulting in stimulation of the parasympathetic pathways and an increase in vagal activity, leading to a fall in the heart rate. The decelerations occur after the

contraction owing to the time it takes for the circulating blood to reach the aortic arch from the placenta. In between the contractions the rate of oxygen transfer between the placenta and the fetus is adequate, and the fetal heart rate baseline and variability are normal, indicating adequate cerebral oxygenation. If, however, the fetus is already compromised, then the reduced amount of oxygen transferred during a contraction may not be sufficient to maintain myocardial activity. Direct myocardial depression occurs, in addition to an increase in vagal activity. The rate of oxygen transfer in between the contractions may not be sufficient to maintain adequate oxygenation, which will be characterised by a decrease, or absence, of variability and, eventually, baseline tachycardia.

Causes. Any condition which causes a reduction in placental blood flow may result in late decelerations, for example:

Placental abruption
Maternal hypotension
Excessive uterine activity.

In addition, any maternal or pregnancy-related disease which may result in placental pathology can also cause late decelerations, for example:

Diabetes mellitus
Pregnancy-induced hypertension
Renal disease.

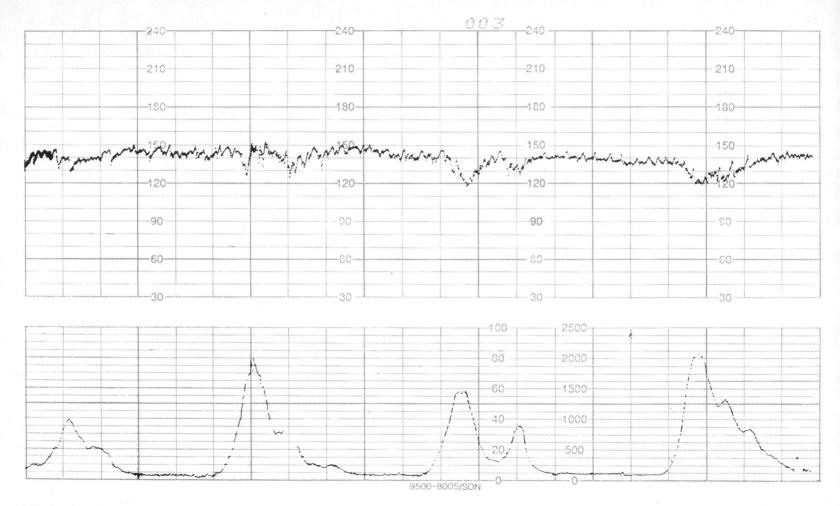

Fig. 3 Early decelerations.

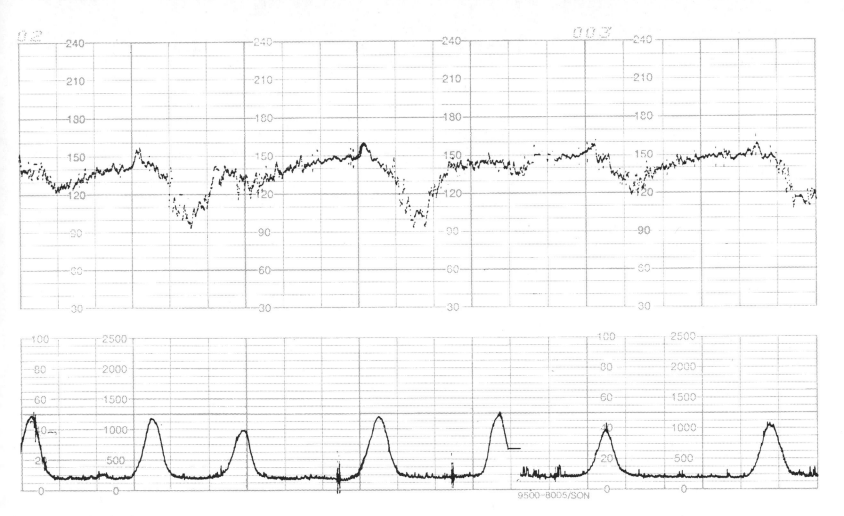

Fig. 4 *Late decelerations.*

Any fetus that is already compromised, either by lack of stored glycogen, or a reduction in circulating red blood cells for the transfer of oxygen, is also at an increased risk of developing late decelerations, Examples of such predisposing circumstances are:

Intrauterine growth retardation
Prematurity
Rhesus isoimmunisation
Twin-to-twin transfusion.

Late decelerations are always associated with significant fetal hypoxia.

Management. The aim is to increase the uterine blood flow and oxygen transfer across the placenta to the fetus.

1. Change maternal posture.
2. Increase or commence intravenous infusion.
3. Give facial oxygen.
4. Stop any oxytocic infusion if in progress.
5. A fetal blood sample should be obtained to assess the pH value and base excess of the fetal blood.
6. Whilst the above actions are being undertaken, the mother should be prepared for delivery, particularly if the variability is decreased or if baseline tachycardia or bradycardia develops in between the decelerations.

Variable decelerations
Definition. Variable decelerations are inconsistent in shape and in their relationship to uterine contractions. They tend to have an amplitude of 40 b.p.m. or more. Accelerations often precede and follow the deceleration. Figure 5 shows an example CTG exhibiting variable decelerations.

Aetiology. Variable decelerations appear to occur as the result of transient compression of the umbilical cord, between the fetus and surrounding maternal tissues or fetal parts, during a uterine contraction.

During a uterine contraction, the venous return is obstructed, leading to a decrease in venous return to the fetal heart. This in turn results in a decrease in cardiac output, and therefore arterial pressure. The baroreceptors in the aortic arch are stimulated and sympathetic activity is increased, resulting in a rise in the fetal heart rate to maintain the blood pressure. With further cord compression, the arterial flow becomes obstructed and fetal hypertension results. The baroreceptors in the aortic arch are stimulated, this time resulting in increased parasympathetic activity leading to a fall in the fetal heart rate, also in an attempt to maintain the blood pressure at a normal level. The deceleration now occurs. As the contraction subsides and the arterial flow obstruction is removed, fetal hypotension recurs until the venous flow returns to normal. A reactionary tachycardia develops. When the contraction has ended, the venous flow returns to normal and the fetal heart rate returns to the baseline.

The effect of variable decelerations upon the fetus varies depending upon the duration and degree of cord occlusion that occurs during a contraction. The longer that the deceleration lasts, and the greater the amplitude, the more suggestive it is of fetal compromise. However, the baseline of the fetal heart and the variability in between the decelerations are the best indicators of fetal oxygenation.

Causes. Variable decelerations are commonly seen when there is any form of umbilical cord entanglement, for example:

Umbilical cord around the neck or body
True knot in the umbilical cord
Prolapsed umbilical cord.

Management. This is aimed at attempting to relieve the cord compression:

1. Change the maternal posture.
2. Vaginal examination to exclude cord prolapse if this is deemed to be a possibility.
3. Stop any oxytocic infusion, if in progress.
4. Increase intravenous fluids.
5. Give facial oxygen.
6. If the decelerations are persistent, severe, or if the variability in between them is reduced, fetal blood sampling should be performed to assess the pH value and base excess of the blood. The mother should be prepared for delivery while this is being performed.

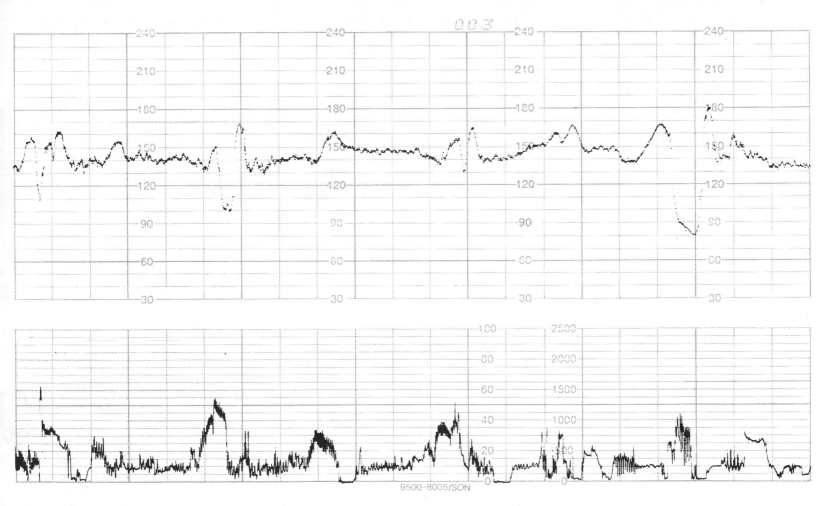

Fig. 5 *Variable decelerations.*

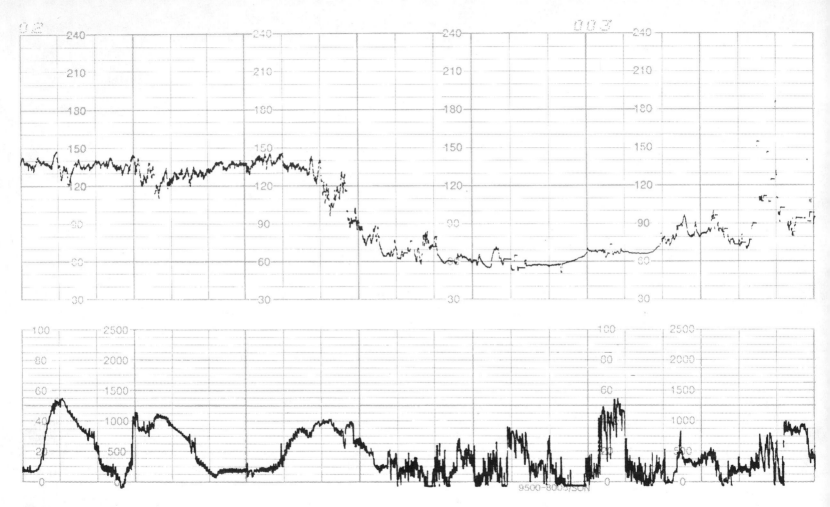

Fig. 6 Prolonged deceleration.

Prolonged deceleration

Definition. A prolonged deceleration is described as consisting of a drop in the fetal heart rate of 30 b.p.m. or more, lasting for a period of at least 2 minutes (for an example CTG, see Fig. 6).

Aetiology. Prolonged decelerations are caused by a decrease in oxygen transfer across the placenta to the fetus, usually as a result of a decrease in uterine blood flow. The chemoreceptors in the aortic arch are stimulated, resulting in an increase in parasympathetic activity and a fall in the fetal heart rate.

Prolonged decelerations are commonly associated with preceding variable decelerations.

Causes.
1. Total umbilical cord occlusion, e.g. cord prolapse.
2. Maternal hypotension resulting from the administration of local anaesthetic via an epidural catheter.
3. Uterine hypertonia.
4. Prolonged decelerations can also be evident following vaginal examination or artificial rupture of the membranes. This could be due to direct pressure being applied onto the fetal head, resulting in pressure on the vagal centre in the brain.

Management. This is aimed at increasing the blood flow to the uterus, and the oxygen transfer across the placenta to the fetus. In addition to ascertaining the cause of the deceleration:

1. Change the maternal posture.
2. Increase intravenous fluids.
3. Stop oxytocic infusion, if in progress.
4. Give facial oxygen.
5. Vaginal examination to exclude cord prolapse.
6. Assess maternal blood pressure, particularly if an epidural block is in progress.
7. Prepare the mother for delivery while the above actions are being performed.
8. Obtain a fetal blood sample on recovery of the fetal heart rate to the baseline to assess the pH value and base excess of the blood. If this is performed during the deceleration, then a transient acidosis will be present, but may not be a true reflection of the degree of fetal hypoxia.

If the CTG has been normal beforehand, a definite cause can be attributed to the deceleration, appropriate management is initiated and the fetal heart rate returns to normal, the fetal outcome is usually good. If the variability is decreased, or any other fetal heart rate abnormalities are present, then this is more suggestive of significant fetal hypoxia.

MANAGEMENT OF FETAL HEART RATE ABNORMALITIES

The management of the periodic changes in the fetal heart rate that have been suggested are aimed at reducing the degree of fetal hypoxia and therefore improving the CTG. The measures, excluding fetal blood sampling, are non-invasive and can be performed quickly.

Medical staff should be informed of any fetal heart rate abnormalities that occur on a CTG. The actions suggested can be performed while waiting for them to attend, in the hope that an improvement in the pattern will be evident before they arrive.

Many single fetal heart rate abnormalities will resolve with conservative management (Grant 1989). In cases where multiple abnormalities are evident, conservative management, whilst preparations are being made to expedite delivery, may not greatly improve the degree of fetal hypoxia.

If the cause of the fetal heart rate abnormality can be ascertained, e.g. late decelerations occurring due to overstimulation of uterine activity with an oxytocic infusion, and the stimulus removed, the fetus is likely to recover more quickly in utero than if it were delivered in a severely hypoxic condition (Cohen & Schifrin 1978).

Attempts should always be made to employ conservative management of fetal heart rate abnormalities, even if a decision has been made to deliver the fetus immediately.

FETAL COMPROMISE

Fetal compromise occurs as a result of an asphyxial insult which gives rise to intrauterine hypoxia. Fetal heart rate abnormalities on a CTG should alert staff to the possibility that some degree of hypoxia exists (Arulkumaran & Chua 1996). Fetal hypoxia develops when insufficient oxygen is transferred from the mother to the fetus through the placenta, or if the transfer of oxygen is adequate, but the fetus is unable to utilise it owing to, for example, impaired circulation.

Throughout pregnancy, the fetus depends upon supplies of glucose and oxygen from the mother, which are necessary for its energy requirements. Some of the glucose is utilised immediately, the remainder being stored in the liver as glycogen, particularly during the third trimester of pregnancy. During labour, when maternal supplies of glucose and oxygen are diminished, and energy requirements raised, the fetus can draw upon these reserves of glycogen. The fetus converts the stored glycogen into acids; then, in the presence of oxygen, into carbon dioxide and water. The carbon dioxide is rapidly disposed of by diffusion across the placenta. This process requires blood flow to be effective. If there is any impairment, i.e. umbilical cord occlusion or placental abruption, the transfer of oxygen and carbon dioxide between the mother and fetus is diminished. This results in a rise in the carbon dioxide levels in the blood of the fetus. Carbonic acid is formed by the hydration of the excess carbon dioxide. Subsequently, a respiratory acidosis develops. The pH value of the blood falls, i.e. becomes more acid, although little change is seen in the acid–base balance or base excess, suggesting that the buffers that exist in the blood to neutralise acids and maintain the pH are still in evidence.

Respiratory acidosis can arise quickly and can also recover quickly if adequate oxygenation is resumed. This involves increasing the uterine blood flow and therefore the rate of transfer of oxygen and carbon dioxide across the placenta.

If respiratory acidosis is not corrected, and the transfer of oxygen to the fetus from the mother is not improved, then insufficient oxygen is available to convert the acids, produced in the metabolism of glycogen, into carbon dioxide and water. The fetus is only able to dispose of these acids by diffusion through the placenta, which is a much slower process than the diffusion of carbon dioxide. Levels of lactic acid accumulate in the fetal circulation, resulting in a metabolic acidosis. The pH value of the blood falls, becoming more acidic, while the acid–base balance or base excess rises, suggesting that the buffers of the blood are being utilised rapidly in an attempt to maintain the pH. The presence of a metabolic acidosis implies that the length and severity of the asphyxial insult that has resulted in hypoxia has been more prolonged than the presence of a respiratory acidosis suggests.

Under normal circumstances, adequate oxygenation of the fetal tissues is maintained by the good uterine blood flow, the high fetal cardiac output and the enhanced oxygen-carrying capacity of the fetal blood. However, in circumstances where the placenta does not function adequately, or placental pathology develops, fetal oxygenation may be impaired, for example in:

Diabetes mellitus
Pregnancy-induced hypertension
Placental abruption
Postmaturity.

The fetus's ability to compensate for hypoxia is also impaired if the glycogen stores are reduced. The fetus is then unable to create sufficient energy from the metabolism of the stores. Examples of such circumstances are:

Prematurity
Intrauterine growth retardation.

Any condition present in the fetus that involves a reduction in the oxygen-carrying capacity of the blood will also lead to a predisposition to developing hypoxia, for example:

Anaemia
Rhesus incompatibility
Twin-to-twin transfusion
Fetal infection when oxygen requirements are raised.

FETAL BLOOD SAMPLING

Fetal heart rate abnormalities arising on a CTG should be considered as an alerting factor to the possibility that the fetus is suffering some degree of hypoxia. However, this is a subjective diagnosis. For the diagnosis to be more accurate, interpretation of the CTG should be combined with fetal blood sampling, and the assessment of the pH value and base excess of the fetal blood. In 1985 MacDonald and colleagues concluded that there was little justification for the use of electronic fetal monitoring without the facilities to assess fetal acid–base status; a view supported by others (Murphy et al 1990, RCOG 1993, Sawers 1983, Van Den Berg et al 1987).

REFERENCES

Arulkumaran S, Chua S 1996 Cardiotocograph in labour. Current Obstetrics and Gynaecology 6(4): 182–188

Cohen W, Schifrin B 1978 Diagnosis and management of fetal distress during labour. Seminars in Perinatology 2(2): 155–167

Grant A 1989 Monitoring the fetus during labour. In: Chalmers I, Enkin M, Keirse M (eds) Effective care in pregnancy and childbirth. Oxford University Press, Oxford, pp 846–888

MacDonald D, Grant A, Sheridan-Pereira M, Boylen P, Chalmers I 1985 The Dublin randomised controlled trial of intrapartum fetal heart rate monitoring. American Journal of Obstetrics and Gynecology 52: 524–539

Murphy K W, Johnston P, Moorcraft J 1990 Birth asphyxia and the intrapartum cardiotocograph. British Journal of Obstetrics and Gynaecology 97(6): 470–479

O'Connor M C, Hassabo M S, McFadyen R 1980 Is the sinusoidal fetal heart rate pattern sinister. Journal of Obstetrics and Gynaecology. 1(2): 90–95

Royal College of Obstetricians and Gynaecologists 1993 26th RCOG Study Group. Intrapartum fetal surveillance. RCOG Press, London

Sawers R S 1983 Fetal monitoring during labour. British Medical Journal 287 (6406): 1649–1650

Van Den Berg P, Schmidt S, Gesch J 1987 Fetal distress and the condition of the newborn using cardiotocography and fetal blood analysis during labour. British Journal of Obstetrics and Gynaecology 94(1): 72–75

Young B K, Katz M, Wilson S J 1980 Sinusoidal fetal heart rate. Clinical significance. American Journal of Obstetrics and Gynecology 136: 587–593

RECOMMENDED RESOURCES

Enkin M, Keirse M J N C, Renfrew M, Neilson J (eds) 1996 Care of the fetus during labour. In: A guide to effective care in pregnancy and childbirth. Oxford University Press, Oxford, ch 30

An excellent resource containing a collection and systematic review of randomised trials in obstetric and midwifery practice. Each chapter ends with a comment by the reviewer on the implications for practice. Also available in an electronic database, The Cochrane Library, updated as reviews occur.

Gibb D, Arulkamaran S 1997 Fetal monitoring in practice, 2nd edn. Butterworth Heinemann, Oxford

Clear and concise book on fetal well-being, heart rate monitoring and techniques. There are helpful explanations of monitoring techniques with illustrations. There is also an exposition of trace analysis with examples offered.

MIDIRS (Midwives Information and Resource Service) and the NHS Centre for Reviews and Dissemination

- *Fetal heart rate monitoring in labour. Informed choice for professionals leaflet*
- *Listening to your baby's heartbeat during labour. Informed choice for mothers leaflet. MIDIRS, Bristol*

These leaflets are based on the best scientific evidence available. There are two leaflets for each topic, one for the professional and one for the mother. Clear, easy to read.

The Cochrane Library, Update Software, Oxford

This is an electronic database of systematic reviews updated as new trials are reported and gives the best available evidence in a number of areas including childbirth. Published in CD-ROM or disk format. Most maternity units have this database which is accessible by midwives and doctors.

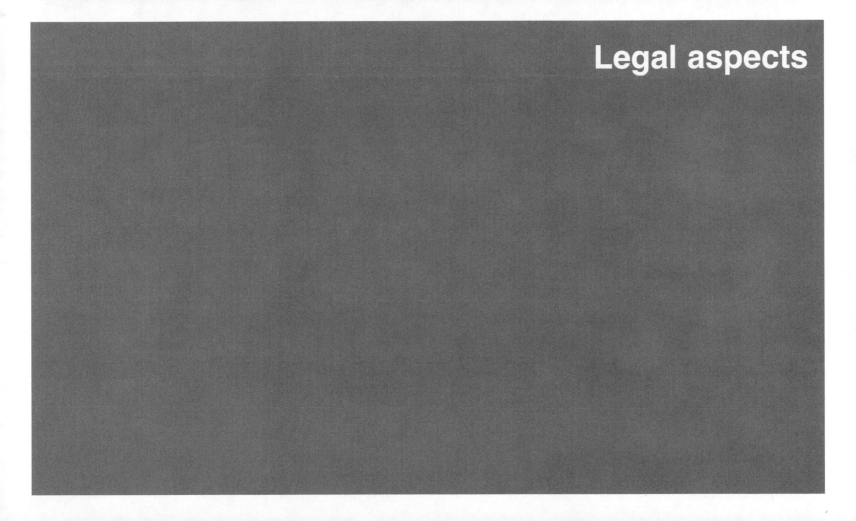

PART 2

Legal aspects

CHAPTER 3

Litigation and risk management

Andrew Symon

INTRODUCTION

This chapter places the importance of cardiotocography within its legal context by examining the relevant literature and using a number of legal cases to illustrate critical areas. It then identifies how risk management tries to reduce the incidence of poor clinical outcomes through the judicious use of the cardiotocograph (CTG) and through encouraging appropriate training and supervision for those who use the CTG.

Risk management in health care relates to any adverse event. Such a wide concept covers many different fields, including clinical competence, and the health and safety of all who enter a hospital. This chapter is only concerned with one very specific aspect of risk management, namely the use of the CTG and its relationship with litigation.

Cardiotocography is an aspect of clinical care which has attracted considerable attention in legal cases, particularly those concerning cerebral palsy. While its level of use may be debated, those doctors and midwives who use this form of monitoring must be adequately trained in its interpretation. Designed as a means of identifying the distressed fetus, the CTG has obvious clinical (as well as medicolegal) implications. Nevertheless, its routine application has been criticised.

BACKGROUND

Electronic fetal monitoring was pioneered in 1958 by Hon, but the first commercially available monitor was not produced until 1968 (Gibb & Arulkumaran 1997). Since then, however, CTG use has grown rapidly. Murphy et al (1990, p. 470) claim that continuous monitoring has become integral to obstetric practice, 'despite the fact that no clear evidence exists for its efficacy, especially in low risk pregnancy.' Their study found a low degree of specificity (i.e. many false positives – staff diagnosing fetal compromise when it did not exist) and they conclude that this is one of the main reasons for current dissatisfaction with this method of monitoring. They stress the need to view the CTG in conjunction with other assessments such as fetal blood sampling (FBS), and not as the sole indicator of the fetal condition. Despite this, the use of FBS varies enormously.

It must be remembered that the CTG is only one marker of possible fetal compromise: its ability to identify with certainty the compromised fetus and so prevent birth asphyxia is therefore limited. The term 'birth asphyxia' is one which, while frequently used, is defined in many different ways. There is no way of measuring asphyxia directly (i.e. measuring oxygen levels in the brain at cellular level), and so indirect measures or markers are used.

These include the CTG, fetal or cord blood pH, or a baby's condition at birth (assessed by the Apgar score) or neurological status in the first few days of life.

Paneth (1993, p. 97) points out that 'The several asphyxial markers do not identify the same infants [so] it is difficult to choose any particular clinical variable as truly representing birth asphyxia … [it] is a research laboratory concept, not yet translatable into a clinical measure.' Because of the difficulties in reaching a comprehensive definition, Blair (1993, p. 449) recommends that 'the term be dropped in clinical practice in favour of terms referring to clinically observable events.' This view has been endorsed by the American College of Obstetricians and Gynecologists (ACOG 1991).

The particular clinical (as well as legal) concern in monitoring a labour is to prevent the hypoxia which can cause damage to brain cells leading to handicap or even death. The condition which has attracted the most attention in this respect is cerebral palsy. Hensleigh et al (1986, p. 979) note that 'the incidence of cerebral palsy in developed countries is about 1.5 to 2.5 per 1000. Comparisons between countries show no correlation with the prevailing perinatal mortality rate.' In other words, intrapartum monitoring measures which were designed to reduce perinatal mortality will have little impact on the incidence of cerebral palsy,

since the factors leading to the two outcomes are apparently different. Stanley (1994) also notes that obstetric technology has done nothing to reduce the incidence of cerebral palsy – indeed, this has increased slightly, a factor attributed to the survival of low-birthweight babies who would not have survived 20 or 30 years ago.

The CTG must be used with caution: it is not the solution to the problem of handicapped infants. When it is used, it must be used for the right reason, and with the appropriate degree of skill. However, some studies have demonstrated considerable difficulties with interpretation of the CTG, including a high degree of false positives and false negatives (Keegan et al 1985), overconfidence in the ability to interpret CTGs (Ennis, unpublished work, 1990), and differences not only between practitioners (Henderson-Smart 1991), but also when the same practitioner examines the same trace twice (Nielsen et al 1987).

With such a low level of agreement about use and interpretation, it is perhaps surprising that the CTG still forms such an integral part of legal wranglings; however, when the issue is a brain-damaged baby, this is often very much the case. Successive Confidential Enquiries into Stillbirths and Deaths in Infancy (e.g. MCHRC 1997) have highlighted the CTG as a significant factor in poor outcomes; and staff deficiencies in CTG use which result in litigation have been identified

by Ennis & Vincent (1990), Capstick & Edwards (1990), James (1991), and Vincent et al (1991).

THE CTG IN LITIGATION

The law regarding clinical negligence is ably covered in standard texts (e.g. Dimond 1994, Payne-James et al 1996), and I do not propose to cover this. The object here is to demonstrate how the CTG has become a feature of litigation. Ennis & Vincent's (1990) study of 64 legal cases found a number of complaints made about CTGs. These included unsatisfactory or missing traces, abnormalities being ignored or not noticed, and traces simply not being done. Of 11 in this category, they note that in three 'midwives were asked by a doctor to carry out CTG but forgot' (p. 1366). The problem of a CTG trace going missing was also noted by James (1991, p. 38): 'The cardiotocograph record is often crucial yet its bulk at the end of a long and complicated labour makes it difficult to store securely within the records. However, claims have become indefensible because this vital piece of evidence was missing, the notes were inadequate, or key personnel could not be traced.'

Capstick & Edwards (1990) identified problems with not noticing signs of fetal distress, or not taking appropriate action quickly when such signs were noticed.

Vincent et al (1991, p. 392) noted that missing or poor quality traces were significant, and also found that interpretation was a recurrent theme: 'In 14 cases the doctor or midwife simply did not recognise an abnormal trace. In five the abnormality was noted, but no action was taken; the staff believed the machine to be faulty and so ignored the trace.'

These features all point to significant deficiencies in staff competence, whether they relate to clinical abilities or communication skills. Such deficiencies are highlighted in the legal journals too (e.g. *Wisniewski v. Central Manchester HA* 1996, *Gaughan v. Bedfordshire HA* 1997, *Dowdie v. Camberwell HA* 1997, *Robertson v. Nottingham HA* 1997), and were in evidence in many of the cases which formed part of a large-scale study into perinatal litigation.* A small selection of these cases is reported

The legal cases referred to (not those reported in the legal journals) come from Scotland and England, and were examined during the course of doctoral research based at the University of Edinburgh, 1993–1997. Funding for this came from the Economic and Social Research Council, the National Board for Nursing, Midwifery and Health Visiting for Scotland, and the Iolanthe Research Fellowship. Study time of 1 day a week was allowed by the Perth and Kinross Healthcare NHS Trust and was invaluable. The success (or otherwise) of these cases should not be inferred from the brief extracts given. The PhD was awarded in July 1997.

here. I have used extracts to illustrate some of the circumstances in which the CTG has become integral to a legal action. These include failing to use the CTG when there is an indication to do so, the inappropriate use of equipment, and poor interpretation of the CTG trace.

When to monitor?
In one of the cases reviewed, there were persistent early fetal heart rate (FHR) decelerations. The midwifery staff appeared to think these were benign, despite there being reduced FHR variability and meconium staining of the liquor. The expert report stated:

'There is a period of 90 minutes … when there was no CTG recording. This is an unacceptable situation where the patient has had a previous section, [is] at 42 weeks with meconium staining, and with CTG abnormalities which are persistent and who was on Oxytocin.' (Case 1)

This catalogue of 'at risk' factors does not appear to have alerted midwives to the need for extra vigilance, and unsurprisingly this case was conceded by the defence. However, given the desire of some pregnant women for minimal monitoring and intervention in labour, the decision to use the CTG is evidently not always automatic, even when certain 'at risk' factors are present. In another case the woman complained that she should have been monitored more closely,

despite having asked in advance of her labour for minimal monitoring. In fact, during labour the CTG had been discontinued at her request owing to discomfort. Her solicitor claimed:

'Continuous fetal monitoring when the decision was made to give a syntocinon infusion should have been insisted upon…' (Case 2)

While many staff would agree that the use of Syntocinon to augment labour is an indication for continuous monitoring by CTG, this case illustrates the balancing act which staff must attempt. There is on the one hand a desire to accede to a specific request (the matter of choice having been given great scope in the 'Changing Childbirth' document (DoH 1993) and the Scottish Policy Review (Scottish Office 1993)), and on the other using clinical judgement and (increasingly) following unit protocols which may contradict the woman's stated preference.

Difficulties with monitoring have been encountered in some cases:

The plaintiffs claimed that monitoring should not have been discontinued. The midwife documented that it was very difficult to listen to the fetal heart as the labouring woman moved and rocked a lot.

The midwife looking after her noted frequent 'loss of contact' on the CTG trace, and stated: 'I made the decision to stop the print out from the monitor but kept the transducer and belt in situ, and I was continually listening to the fetal heart.' (Case 3)

The midwives' reports indicated that the fetal heart rate was satisfactory at all times, but there is clearly a difficulty in situations like this. When a probe must be held in position in order to hear the fetal heart rate clearly, writing contemporaneous entries in the woman's case notes is impossible. A midwife's responsibility is to ensure that she completes the notes as soon as she can. It may be that having notepaper to hand, and writing times and heart rates down as an 'aide-mémoire' would help.

Using the equipment correctly
In another legal case the plaintiff's solicitors claimed:

'It would appear that a foetal monitor was incorrectly adjusted and, accordingly, the readings which it gave were not properly interpreted and significant abnormalities were disregarded.' (Case 4)

The CTG had 'wrong speed' written on it. It transpired that different speeds were used at different times in labour, and no times were logged, so the trace was more difficult to interpret. (The case occurred a number of years ago; more modern CTG machines automatically print the date and time on the trace regularly.)

There have been times when the CTG machine itself appears to cause problems:

The plaintiff's solicitors claimed that instead of diagnosing fetal distress in labour, staff assumed the 'heart rate coming and going' was due to a defective CTG machine. Only when the third machine (they claim) was showing the same sort of trace was the woman sent for caesarean section. There is nothing documented to say the CTG machine was replaced at all. Eventually the CTG traces were found, and they revealed one change of machine, from an old to a new model. (Case 5)

The fact that equipment is defective is no defence. In this case there was a gap of $2\frac{1}{2}$ hours when the CTG was not on. There were six written recordings of a fetal heart rate during this period, at half-hourly intervals. The expert report criticised the midwives for not having a more detailed record. Documentation is discussed later in the chapter (p. 36).

Interpretation of the trace
It seems obvious to state that staff who use CTGs must be able to interpret them, but sadly this ability is lacking all too often. In one case the expert report stated:

'I do not recall having ever seen a trace with such a smooth line and almost complete lack of beat to beat variation … The nursing [sic] staff faithfully recorded the events but apparently failed to appreciate the significance of the flat

trace and therefore did not report it to the medical staff.' (Case 4)

There are other cases in which the CTG has shown abnormalities which were ignored by staff. In one instance the expert reported:

'It is difficult to see the point of fetal monitoring if no action is to be taken when there are obvious abnormalities in the recording.' (Case 6)

Staff must be educated and trained in order to make an intelligent interpretation of CTG traces. However, all too frequently it must be questioned whether staff are adequately prepared for this part of their work. In another case a junior midwife was heavily criticised:

The defence solicitor stated: '(The midwife) admitted quite freely that she spent many hours in watching a fetal heart monitor which she was insufficiently trained to interpret or understand at the time. She has since been better trained and, looking back at the fetal heart traces during the period she was on duty, she sees them as being abnormal. In my opinion, quite a bit of liability must therefore attach to a system which asked midwives to watch a monitor which they are insufficiently trained to understand.' (Case 7)

All staff, of whatever grade, must be trained in CTG interpretation if they are called upon to use the technology. Ennis & Vincent (1990) note that in some of the legal cases which they analysed, midwives had correctly noted a fetal heart rate abnormality, but this was ignored by the doctor. In some of the cases of litigation referred to above it was seen that midwives had failed to notify the medical staff despite ominous traces. Clearly there are differences of opinion at times. Such differences were highlighted in related research (Symon 1998) which examined the views of a large number of midwives and obstetricians concerning litigation and certain related aspects.

In this research one doctor commented that: 'Overdiagnosis of "distress" is a large problem.'

From the midwife's point of view there came this comment: 'It can be very frustrating for midwives to inform doctors of a suspected abnormality, to have it ignored before client, and to have to repeatedly call the doctor back.'

Such differences of opinion must be addressed, and it is one of the aims of risk management to do this.

RISK MANAGEMENT

As stated in the introduction to the chapter, risk management covers many different areas, even within maternity care. Although the previous section examined the role of the CTG in litigation, it should not be concluded that risk management aims only to minimise potential exposure to litigation (although this is of course one of its aims).

Clinical risk management aims to minimise the incidence of adverse outcomes, and to facilitate effective claims management by establishing early client contact, and ensuring that all relevant documents are completed (Dineen 1996). While there may be some debate as to what exactly constitutes an adverse outcome, it is clear that the perception of the woman concerned (and possibly that of her family) is crucial. Within this there is a considerable literature about expectations and experiences (see list of Further reading, p. 39). Simply put, some believe that health service practitioners have contributed to these high (sometimes unrealistic) expectations and to consequent dissatisfaction with a less than ideal outcome (cf. Ranjan 1993, Symon 1998).

Within obstetrics and midwifery – and in terms of risk management we must concede that perinatal care is a multidisciplinary field – there are several areas which can be targeted from a risk management point of view. Its interdependence with audit has been stressed (Beard & O'Connor 1995), as has the importance of effective communication between doctors and midwives (James 1991). Documentation is also a critical area: without a detailed (and legible) account of the events in question it may be impossible to determine whether a particular outcome might have been prevented, and whether the appropriate lessons will be learned.

Training and supervision

It is essential that staff who are called upon to interpret CTG traces are competent to do so. In-service education is the standard means of ensuring this (Murphy et al (1990) call for this to be mandatory), but it was worrying to find in a large-scale survey of obstetricians and midwives (Symon 1998) that 65% of the obstetricians felt that training for midwives was deficient in this regard, and that many midwives agreed with this. This must be a matter for concern, for it is the midwife who will usually first pick up on possible problems. The legal (and emotional) consequences of failing to do so may be devastating.

As part of a checklist for risk reduction Drife (1995, p. 139) suggests 'regular training sessions on fetal monitoring' for midwives. This is a minimum requirement: if attendance at a fire lecture can be mandatory in an attempt to reduce risk, then regular in-service training sessions on CTG use and interpretation must be mandatory for practitioners who use this technology. Differences of opinion over interpretation will continue to occur, but can be reduced by the thorough education of staff regarding the use *and limitations* of the CTG. As discussed in the Background section at the beginning of this chapter, the CTG is only one marker of the fetal condition.

With regard to competence, the UKCC Code of Professional Conduct (1992) 'encourages (practitioners) to declare their incompetence in certain procedures rather than to try to undertake them.' While employers have a duty to provide training for their staff, individual midwives also have a responsibility to ensure that they are adequately prepared for the duties entrusted to them, and to request supervision where necessary.

New staff – especially newly qualified staff – must be supervised until their competence is assured (Case 7 above makes this point). Competence cannot be assumed simply because someone has been in post for a few weeks or months. In this regard locum or agency staff present a particular problem: although qualified, their competence and skill may not have been demonstrated in that particular unit. Beard & O'Connor (1995) recommend that full supervision by a member of the regular staff be carried out. For medical staff this may be effected by introducing dedicated consultant sessions in the labour ward – a move supported by the Royal College of Obstetricians and Gynaecologists.

Communication
Drife (1995, p. 139) goes on to call for 'clear definition of (the midwife's) role vis-a-vis SHOs'. If midwives are competent in interpreting CTG traces, but cannot (for whatever reason) communicate this to the medical staff, then there is a problem. Drife (p. 134) acknowledges that the hierarchy

within a hospital can cause difficulties: 'A midwife may be frustrated by a doctor who does not respond appropriately to her concerns: yet she may be reluctant to "go over the head" of a junior doctor to a more senior doctor.'

Beard & O'Connor (1995) also note that the sharing of care between doctor and midwife can be problematic: 'Experience has shown that risk is increased if a midwife retains care for too long, or if a doctor, out of ignorance or faulty decision making, fails to accept responsibility for such a case.' In a situation like this it is imperative that practitioners communicate effectively. Good relationships may be helped through setting up an informal forum for the discussion of particular cases. Such an initiative must at all costs avoid becoming a 'finger-pointing' exercise: that would destroy any hope of the mutual respect which underpins effective communication.

Communication between staff and the labouring woman, and (where appropriate) her family, is vital too: Dillner (1995) notes the role of poor communication in suboptimal outcomes. Monitoring can only be carried out with the woman's consent, and this may be difficult to obtain if she is in pain or upset because of events, or is under the effects of opiate or inhalational analgesia.

Equipment
While it may be tempting to assume that equipment within maternity units is efficient

and well maintained, in view of the legal cases concerning apparently defective machinery, this is not a safe assumption. Obsolete monitors must be replaced, and those which are used maintained to an acceptable standard. This of course has cost implications, but must be more financially appealing than the prospect of paying out hundreds of thousands of pounds because monitoring was either deficient or not carried out at all.

Because the CTG is only one marker of the fetal condition, it is recommended that equipment for fetal blood sampling also be provided (Drife 1995, Murphy et al 1990).

Documentation
This aspect of care has been highlighted by many authors (e.g. Cetrulo & Cetrulo 1989, James 1991, McRae 1993), especially with regard to potential litigation. Cohn (1984, p. 321) notes that 'good record keeping is the single most useful thing that can be done to minimize risk, other than to talk with and take good care of patients.'

The CTG trace is part of the clinical documentation, and is therefore a legal document. However, a particular difficulty with the CTG is storage. Bear in mind that many legal actions are not raised for several years (in cases involving cerebral palsy there is effectively no time limit), and because the paper on which traces are printed is heat and light sensitive, and liable to tearing, it must be protected securely. Some units have introduced a sturdy envelope (for CTG traces only) which can be attached inside the case notes.

Because missing or deficient CTG traces have been a particular problem in litigation, it is vital that midwives also record the fetal heart rate in the woman's case notes. Entries relating to rate and variability, as well as accelerations and decelerations, will help to clarify the record of this important marker of the fetal condition in the event that the CTG trace is unavailable. These entries should be made in the notes as soon as possible: any delay decreases the likelihood that staff will be able to recall accurately a sequence of events and results. Failing to make any entries for long periods can leave the impression that the women was unsupervised (not an uncommon allegation), and can give the impression that care was substandard. This is best summed up by the adage 'If you didn't write it, you didn't do it.'

CONCLUSION

All the suggestions made here may seem obvious. However, reflecting a point made by Cohn (1984), if the problems caused by failing to implement these points were rare, they would not be cited here. Many poor outcomes (and subsequent legal cases) simply would not arise if these points were taken on board and implemented effectively. However, we do not live in an ideal world: staff will have 'off days', communication with colleagues and with women and their families may be difficult, and pressure of work may leave little time for writing in the case notes.

CTGs, however, remain a critical part of intrapartum care, and constitute a significant factor in litigation. Risk management in this respect is the responsibility both of employers and of individual practitioners. There is no magic wand which will make these problems go away, and while obvious, the suggestions for effective risk management require the support and cooperation of all grades of clinical staff and their managers.

REFERENCES

American College of Obstetricians and Gynecologists (ACOG) 1991 Utility of umbilical cord blood acid–base assessment. Committee on Obstetrics, Maternal and Fetal Medicine of the American College of Obstetricians and Gynecologists: ACOG Committee Opinion #91

Beard R, O'Connor A 1995 Implementation of audit and risk management: a protocol. In: Vincent C (ed) Clinical risk management. BMJ Publishing Group, London, pp 350–374

Blair E 1993 A research definition for 'birth asphyxia'? Developmental Medicine and Child Neurology 35: 449–455

Capstick J B, Edwards P 1990 Trends in obstetric malpractice claims. Lancet 336: 931–932

Cetrulo C, Cetrulo L 1989 The legal liability of the medical consultant in pregnancy. Medical Clinics of North America 73(3): 557–565

Cohn S 1984 The nurse–midwife: malpractice and risk management. Journal of Nurse–Midwifery 29: 316–321

Department of Health 1993 Changing childbirth: report of the Expert Maternity Group. HMSO, London

Dillner L 1995 Babies' deaths linked to suboptimal care. British Medical Journal 310: 757

Dimond B 1994 The legal aspects of midwifery. Books for Midwives Press, Hale

Dineen M 1996 Clinical risk management – a pragmatic approach. British Journal of Midwifery 4: 586–589

Dowdie v. Camberwell Health Authority [1997] 8 Medical Law Reports: 368–376

Drife J O 1995 Risk reduction in obstetrics. In: Vincent C (ed) Clinical risk management. BMJ Publishing Group, London

Ennis M, Vincent C A 1990 Obstetric accidents: a review of 64 cases. British Medical Journal 300: 1365–1367

Gibb D, Arulkumaran S 1997 Fetal monitoring in practice, 2nd edn. Butterworth Heinemann, Oxford

Gaughan v. Bedfordshire Health Authority [1997] 8 Medical Law Reports: 182–190

Henderson-Smart D 1991 Throwing the baby out with the fetal monitoring? Medical Journal of Australia 154: 576–578

Hensleigh P, Fainstat T, Spencer R 1986 Perinatal events and cerebral palsy. American Journal of Obstetrics and Gynecology 154: 978–981

James C 1991 Risk management in obstetrics and gynaecology. Journal of the Medical Defence Union 7: 36–38

Keegan K, Waffarn F, Quilligan E 1985 Obstetric characteristics and FHR patterns of infants during the newborn period. American Journal of Obstetrics and Gynecology 153: 732–737

McRae M 1993 Litigation, electronic fetal monitoring, and the obstetric nurse. Journal of Obstetric, Gynecological and Neonatal Nursing 22(5): 410–419

Maternal and Child Health Research Consortium (MCHRC) 1997 Confidential enquiry into stillbirths and deaths in infancy. MCHRC, London

Murphy K, Johnson P, Moorcraft J, Pattinson J, Russell V, Turnbull A 1990 Birth asphyxia and the intrapartum cardiotocograph. British Journal of Obstetrics and Gynaecology 97: 470–479

Nielsen P, Stigsby B, Nickelsen C, Nim J 1987 Intra- and inter-observer variability in the assessment of intrapartum CTGs. Acta Obstetrica Gynecologia Scandinavica 66: 421–424

Paneth N 1993 The causes of cerebral palsy: recent evidence. Clinical Investigations in Medicine (Canada) 16: 95–102

Payne-James J, Dean P, Wall I 1996 Medicolegal essentials in healthcare. Churchill Livingstone, New York

Ranjan V 1993 Obstetrics and the fear of litigation. Professional Care of Mother and Child (Jan): 10–12

Robertson v Nottingham Health Authority (1997) 8 Medical Law Reports: 1–15

Scottish Office 1993 The provision of maternity services in Scotland: a policy review. Scottish Office Home and Health Department, Edinburgh

Stanley F 1994 Cerebral palsy – the courts catch up with sad realities. Medical Journal of Australia 161: 236

Symon A 1998 Litigation – the views of midwives and obstetricians. Hochland and Hochland, Hale, Cheshire

United Kingdom Central Council for Nursing, Midwifery and Health Visiting (UKCC) 1992 Code of professional conduct, 3rd edn. UKCC, London

Vincent C, Martin T, Ennis M 1991 Obstetric accidents: the patient's perspective. British Journal of Obstetrics and Gynaecology 98: 390–395

Wisniewski v Central Manchester Health Authority (1996) 7 Medical Law Reports: 248–265

Harpwood V 1996 Legal Issues in obstetrics. Dartmouth, Aldershot

O'Meara C 1993 An evaluation of consumer perspectives of childbirth and parenting education. Midwifery 9: 210–219

Reynolds J, Yudkin P, Bull M 1987 General practitioner obstetrics: does risk prediction work? Journal of the Royal College of General Practitioners 38: 307–310

Spencer J 1993 Clinical overview of cardiotocography. British Journal of Obstetrics and Gynaecology 100 (suppl 9): 4–7

Stanley F, Blair E 1991 Why have we failed to reduce the frequency of cerebral palsy? Medical Journal of Australia 154: 623–626

FURTHER READING

Avis M, Bond M, Arthur A 1997 Questioning patient satisfaction: an empirical investigation in two out-patient clinics. Social Science and Medicine 44: 85–92

Beaton J, Gupton A 1990 Childbirth expectations: a qualitative analysis. Midwifery 6: 133–139

Beech B 1992 Penalties of obstetric technology. 2nd International Homebirth Conference. AIMS Publications, Iver, Bucks

Dingwall R 1991 Risk management. British Medical Journal 302: 255

Case studies

Normal

LIVERPOOL JOHN MOORES UNIVERSITY
LEARNING SERVICES

HISTORY

26-year-old gravida II, para I

Past history
Nil relevant

Antenatal period
Normal
Admitted at 40 weeks with contractions

Labour

09.00 hours
Cervical os 3–4 cm dilated
Artificial rupture of membranes – clear liquor draining
Fetal scalp electrode applied
Intrauterine pressure catheter inserted

09.35 hours
Epidural analgesia commenced

12.00 hours
Cervix 7 cm dilated
CTG

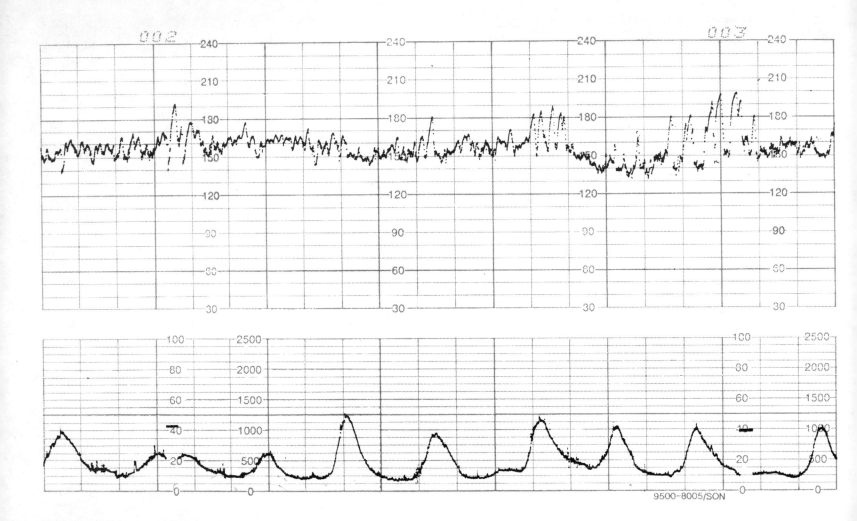

CTG

1 What do you notice about the baseline?

2 What do you notice about the baseline variability?

3 What type of decelerations, if any, are present?

4 What do you notice about the uterine activity?

5 What is the most probable cause of fetal heart rate abnormality shown on this trace?

6 What treatment and/or intervention would you consider necessary for this fetal heart rate pattern?

NOTES

1

2

3

4

5

6

ANALYSIS

1 Baseline 150–155 b.p.m.

2 Variability 5–15 b.p.m.

3 No decelerations, some accelerations

4 Contracting 4 in 10 minutes, varying in strength

5 Normal CTG

6 No action necessary

OUTCOME

13.30 hours
Second stage of labour diagnosed

17.15 hours
Spontaneous vertex delivery
Live girl
Apgar score 9/1 9/5
Birthweight 2.260 kg

HISTORY

23-year-old gravida II, para 0 + 1

Past history
Nil relevant

Antenatal period
Treated for urinary tract infection at 28 weeks
Admitted at 40 weeks with contractions

Labour

15.30 hours
Cervical os 2 cm dilated
Artificial rupture of membranes – clear liquor draining
Fetal scalp electrode applied
Intrauterine pressure catheter inserted

16.05 hours
Epidural analgesia commenced

17.45 hours
CTG

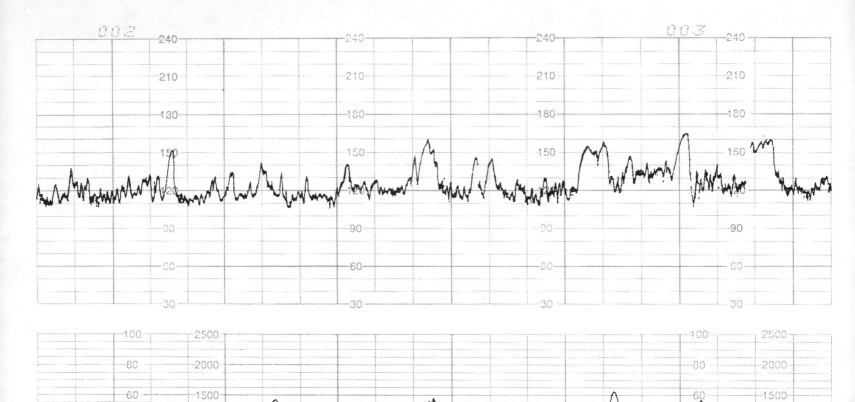

9500-8005/SON

CTG

1 What do you notice about the baseline?

2 What do you notice about the baseline variability?

3 What type of decelerations, if any, are present?

4 What do you notice about the uterine activity?

5 What is the most probable cause of fetal heart rate abnormality shown on this trace?

6 What treatment and/or intervention would you consider necessary for this fetal heart rate pattern?

NOTES

1

2

3

4

5

6

ANALYSIS

1 Baseline 110–120 b.p.m.

2 Variability 5–15 b.p.m.

3 No decelerations, accelerations with some contractions

4 Contracting 4–5 in 10 minutes, varying in strength

5 Normal CTG

6 No action necessary

OUTCOME

04.00 hours
Progressed to second stage of labour

06.00 hours
No progress made
Caesarean section performed
Live boy
Apgar score 9/1 9/5
Birthweight 4.010 kg

3

HISTORY

25-year-old gravida III, para I + I

Past history
Nil relevant

Antenatal period
Twin pregnancy diagnosed on booking scan
Admitted at 37 weeks with spontaneous
rupture of membranes and contractions

Labour

04.00 hours
Cervical os 4 cm dilated
Clear liquor draining
Fetal scalp electrode applied to twin I (faint
line on CTG)
Twin II monitored externally (darker line on
CTG)
Contractions monitored externally

04.50 hours
Epidural analgesia commenced

06.00 hours
Cervical os 6 cm dilated

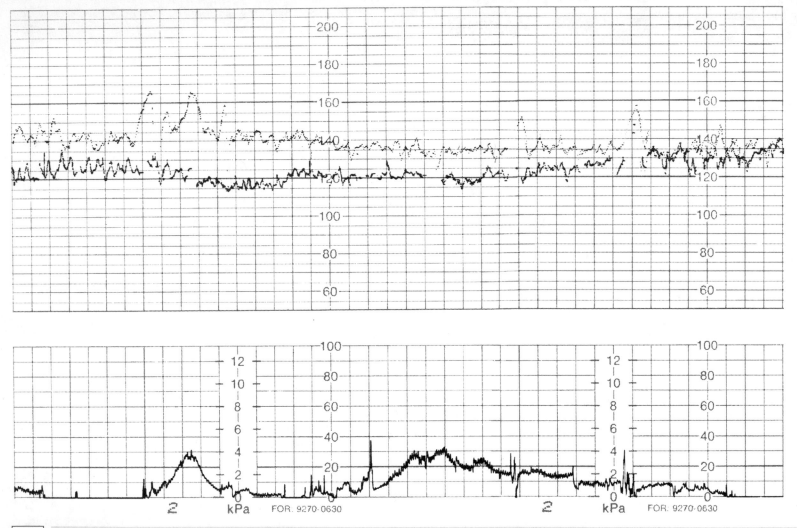

FOR. 9270-0630

FOR. 9270-0630

CTG

1 What do you notice about the baseline?

2 What do you notice about the baseline variability?

3 What type of decelerations, if any, are present?

4 What do you notice about the uterine activity?

5 What is the most probable cause of fetal heart rate abnormality shown on this trace?

6 What treatment and/or intervention would you consider necessary for this fetal heart rate pattern?

NOTES

1

2

3

4

5

6

ANALYSIS

1 Baseline
   Twin I: 130–145 b.p.m.
   Twin II: 115–120 b.p.m.

2 Variability
   Twin I: 5–10 b.p.m.
   Twin II: external, therefore not accurate;
   appears 5–10 b.p.m.

3 No decelerations

4 Contractions not monitored adequately

5 Normal CTG

6 Contractions should be monitored
   No other action necessary

OUTCOME

10.35 hours
Progressed to second stage of labour

12.06 hours
Straight forceps delivery of twin I
Live girl
Apgar score 9/1 9/5
Birthweight 2.470 kg

12.20 hours
Straight forceps delivery of twin II
Live girl
Apgar score 8/1 9/5
Birthweight 2.560 kg

CASE STUDY

30-year-old gravida II, para 1

Past history
Nil relevant

Antenatal period
Progressed normally
Admitted at 41 weeks' plus 2 days' gestation
in spontaneous labour

Labour

03.20 hours
Cervical os 7 cm dilated
Clear liquor draining
Requesting epidural analgesia

3.40 hours
Epidural analgesia commenced
Continuous external monitoring in progress

0430 hours
CTG

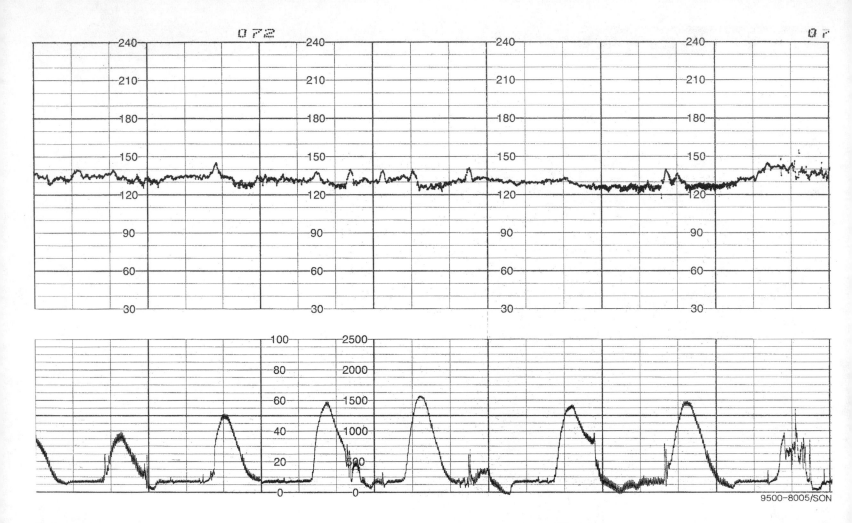

9500−8005/SON

CTG

1 What do you notice about the baseline?

2 What do you notice about the baseline variability?

3 What type of decelerations, if any, are present?

4 What do you notice about the uterine activity?

5 What is the most probable cause of fetal heart rate abnormality shown on this trace?

6 What treatment and/or intervention would you consider necessary for this fetal heart rate pattern?

NOTES

1

2

3

4

5

6

ANALYSIS

1 Baseline 130–135 b.p.m.

2 Variability around 5, acceleration present

3 No decelerations

4 Contracting 3–4 in 10 minutes

5 Normal CTG

6 No action necessary

OUTCOME

Progressed to second stage of labour

09.58 hours
Normal delivery
Live boy
Apgar score 9/1 9/5
Birthweight 3.58 kg

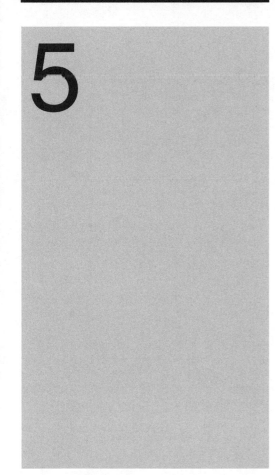

HISTORY

29-year-old gravida II, para I

Past history
Nil relevant

Antenatal period
Twin pregnancy diagnosed on booking scan
Admitted at 36 weeks with contractions

Labour

03.10 hours
Cervical os 4 cm dilated
Artificial rupture of membranes – clear liquor draining
Fetal scalp electrode applied to twin I (faint line on CTG)
Twin II externally monitored (darker line on CTG)
Contractions monitored externally

03.50 hours
Epidural analgesia commenced

08.30 hours
Cervical os 8 cm dilated
CTG

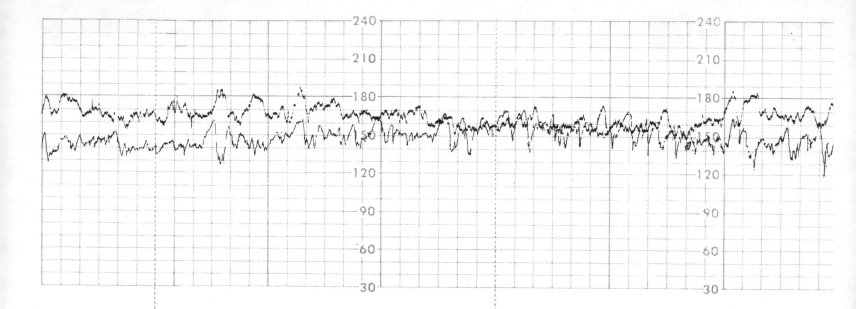
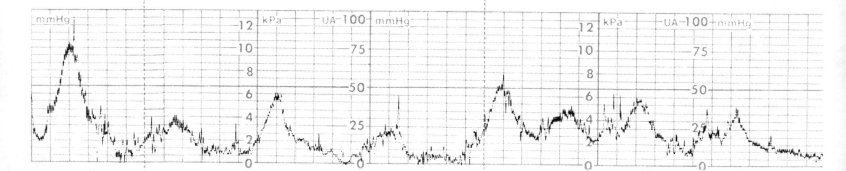

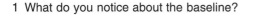

CTG	NOTES
1 What do you notice about the baseline?	1
2 What do you notice about the baseline variability?	
3 What type of decelerations, if any, are present?	2
4 What do you notice about the uterine activity?	3
5 What is the most probable cause of fetal heart rate abnormality shown on this trace?	4
6 What treatment and/or intervention would you consider necessary for this fetal heart rate pattern?	5
	6

ANALYSIS

1 Baseline
   Twin I: 145–150 b.p.m.
   Twin II: 155–165 b.p.m.

2 Variability
   Twin I: 5–10 b.p.m.
   Twin II: external, therefore not accurate;
   appears 5–10 b.p.m.

3 No decelerations

4 Contracting 3–4 in 10 minutes

5 Normal CTG of both twins

6 No action necessary

OUTCOME

09.50 hours
Second stage of labour diagnosed

11.30 hours
Spontaneous vertex delivery of twin I
Live boy
Apgar score 9/1 9/5
Birthweight 2.500 kg

12.20 hours
Straight forceps delivery of twin II
Live boy
Apgar score 9/1 9/5
Birthweight 2.580 kg

HISTORY

20-year-old gravida I, para 0

Past history
Nil relevant

Antenatal period
Normal
Admitted at 40 weeks with contractions

Labour

05.30 hours
Cervical os 5 cm dilated
Artificial rupture of membranes – clear liquor draining
Fetal scalp electrode applied
Intrauterine pressure catheter inserted

06.45 hours
Pethidine 100 mg and Sparine 25 mg given intramuscularly
CTG

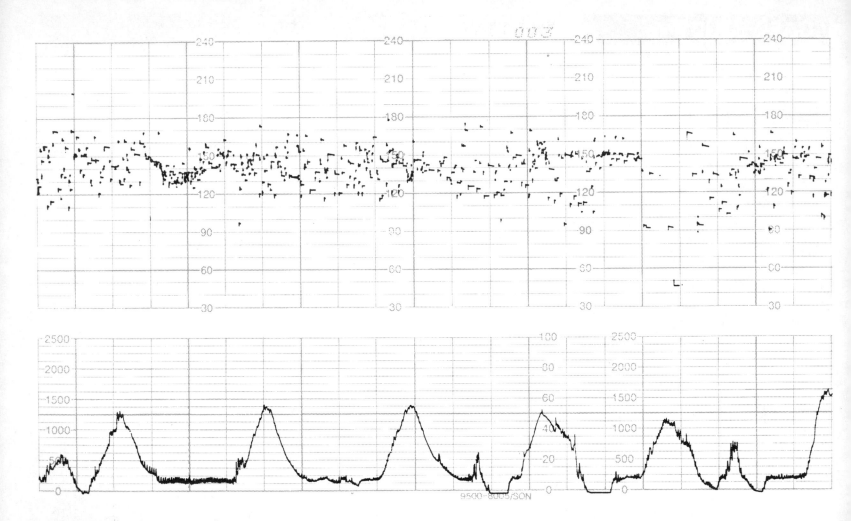

CTG

1 What do you notice about the baseline?

2 What do you notice about the baseline variability?

3 What type of decelerations, if any, are present?

4 What do you notice about the uterine activity?

5 What is the most probable cause of fetal heart rate abnormality shown on this trace?

6 What treatment and/or intervention would you consider necessary for this fetal heart rate pattern?

NOTES

1

2

3

4

5

6

ANALYSIS

Impossible to interpret CTG owing to poor quality print-out.

6 If fetal scalp electrode not working, monitor externally or use intermittent auscultation. The fetal heart rate should be recorded on the CTG.

OUTCOME

13.00 hours
Progressed to second stage of labour

14.25 hours
Spontaneous vertex delivery
Live boy
Apgar score 9/1 9/5
Birthweight 3.250 kg

HISTORY

24-year-old gravida II, para 1

Past history
Nil relevant

Antenatal period
Normal
Admitted at 40 weeks with spontaneous
rupture of membranes and contractions

Labour

10.30 hours
Cervical os 5 cm dilated
Clear liquor draining
Fetal scalp electrode applied
Contractions monitored externally.
Transcutaneous nerve stimulation (TNS) for
analgesia
CTG

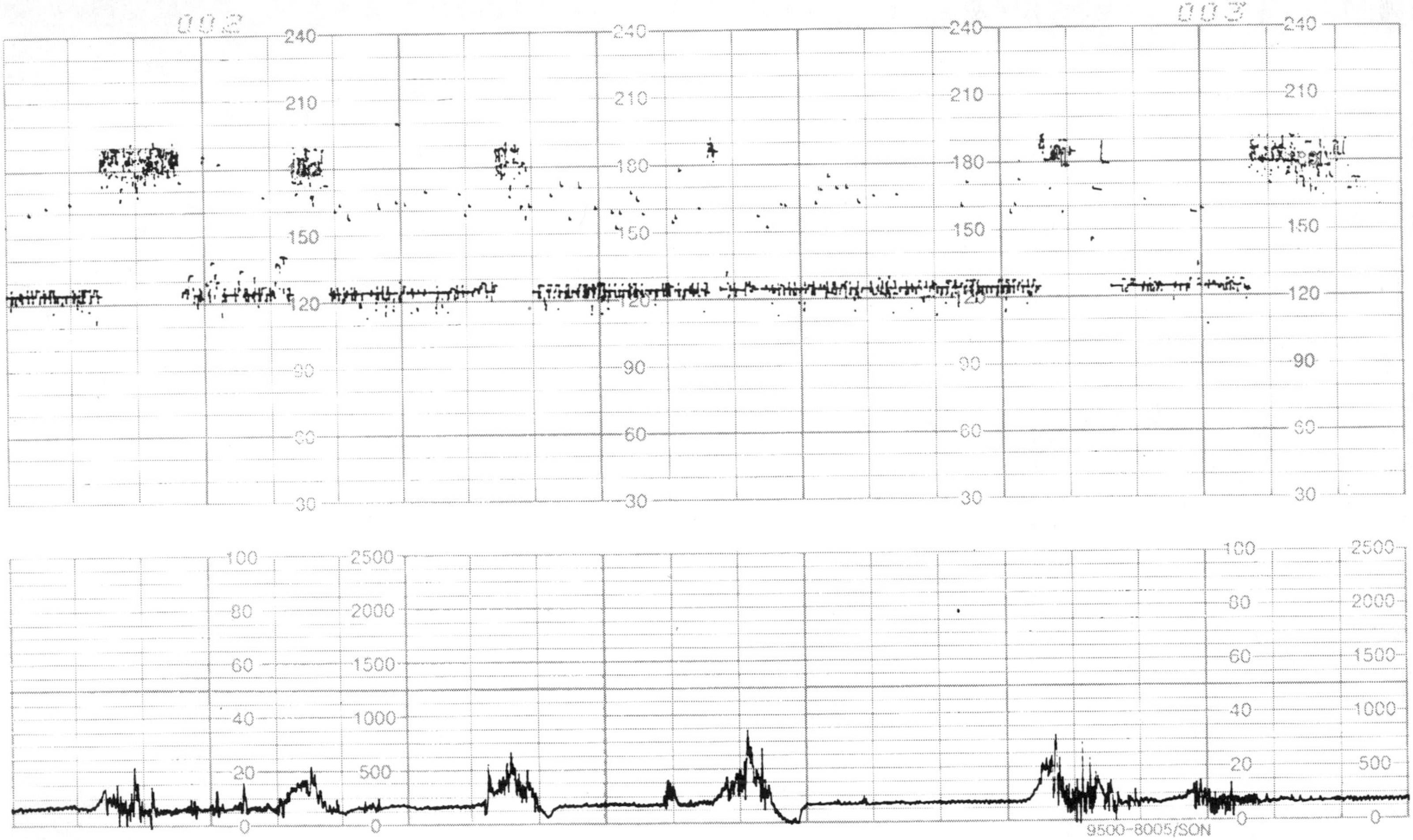
002
003
240
210
180
150
120
90
60
30
100
80
60
40
20
0
2500
2000
1500
1000
500
0
9500-8005/SON

CTG

1 What do you notice about the baseline?

2 What do you notice about the baseline variability?

3 What type of decelerations, if any, are present?

4 What do you notice about the uterine activity?

5 What is the most probable cause of fetal heart rate abnormality shown on this trace?

6 What treatment and/or intervention would you consider necessary for this fetal heart rate pattern?

NOTES

1

2

3

4

5

6

ANALYSIS

Impossible to interpret this CTG, owing to electrical interference from TNS

6 Fetal heart should be auscultated and rate written on CTG
Because of the limited value of the CTG, it is probably better to discontinue it and rely on intermittent auscultation of the fetal heart

OUTCOME

12.30 hours
Second stage of labour diagnosed

12.50 hours
Spontaneous vertex delivery
Live girl
Apgar score 9/1 9/5
Birthweight 3.560 kg

Early decelerations

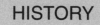
HISTORY

28-year-old gravida IV, para II + I

Past history
Nil relevant

Antenatal period
Normal
Admitted at 41 weeks for surgical induction of labour

Labour

12.45 hours
Cervix 1 cm long, cervical os 1.5 cm dilated
Artificial rupture of membranes – clear liquor draining
Fetal scalp electrode applied
Intrauterine pressure catheter inserted
Syntocinon infusion commenced

15.00 hours
Cervical os 3–4 cm dilated

15.50 hours
Epidural analgesia commenced

17.00 hours
Cervical os 4–5 cm dilated
Syntocinon infusing at 8 mU/min

17.50 hours
CTG

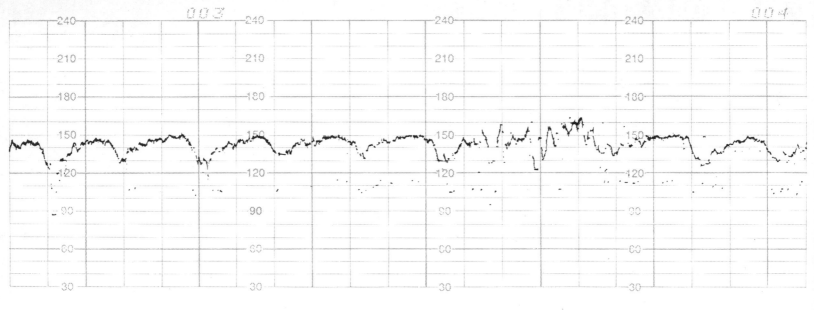

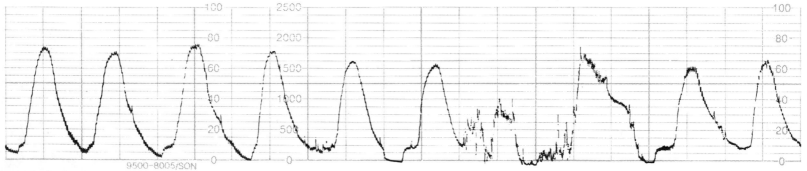

9500-8005/SON

CTG

1 What do you notice about the baseline?

2 What do you notice about the baseline variability?

3 What type of decelerations, if any, are present?

4 What do you notice about the uterine activity?

5 What is the most probable cause of fetal heart rate abnormality shown on this trace?

6 What treatment and/or intervention would you consider necessary for this fetal heart rate pattern?

NOTES

1

2

3

4

5

6

ANALYSIS

1 Baseline 145–150 b.p.m.

2 Variability less than 5 b.p.m.

3 Early decelerations

4 Contracting 5 in 10 minutes, lasting 90
  seconds on average

5 Head compression

6 Change maternal position
  In view of strength and frequency of
  contractions, reduce Syntocinon infusion
  Continue to observe trace for further
  abnormalities

OUTCOME

18.30 hours
Cervical os 9 cm dilated
Syntocinon infusion reduced to 4 mU/min

20.00 hours
Second stage of labour diagnosed

20.30 hours
Commenced pushing
Developed variable decelerations

21.37 hours
Straight forceps delivery for delay in second
stage
Live boy
Apgar score 9/1 10/5
Birthweight 3.870 kg
Cord around neck × 1

HISTORY

21-year-old gravida II, para 0

Past history
Nil relevant

Antenatal period
Normal
Admitted at 42 weeks in spontaneous labour,
contracting 1 in 6 minutes
Cervical os 2–3 cm dilated

21.30 hours
Transferred to ward

Labour

08.00 hours
Cervical os 4 cm dilated
Artificial rupture of membranes – clear liquor
draining
Fetal scalp electrode applied
Intrauterine pressure catheter inserted

11.00 hours
Cervical os 6 cm dilated

11.50 hours
Epidural analgesia commenced

13.30 hours
Cervical os 9 cm dilated

15.00 hours
CTG

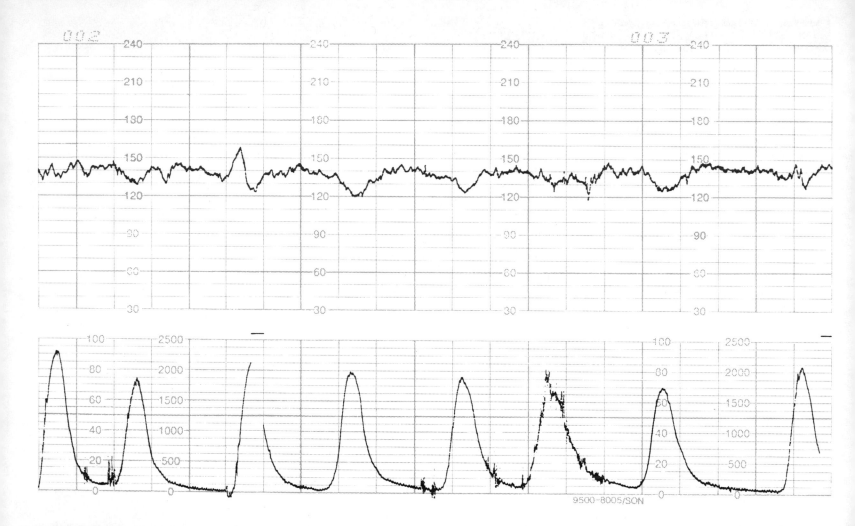

9500-8005/SON

CTG

1 What do you notice about the baseline?

2 What do you notice about the baseline variability?

3 What type of decelerations, if any, are present?

4 What do you notice about the uterine activity?

5 What is the most probable cause of fetal heart rate abnormality shown on this trace?

6 What treatment and/or intervention would you consider necessary for this fetal heart rate pattern?

NOTES

1

2

3

4

5

6

ANALYSIS

1 Baseline 140–145 b.p.m.

2 Variability 5 b.p.m.

3 Early decelerations

4 Contracting 4 in 10 minutes, lasting 90
seconds

5 Head compression

6 Change maternal position
Observe CTG for further abnormalities

OUTCOME

15.55 hours
Second stage of labour diagnosed

16.55 hours
Commenced pushing

17.45 hours
No progress made
Straight forceps delivery
Live boy
Apgar score 9/1 9/5
Birthweight 4.040 kg

HISTORY

24-year-old gravida II, para 0 + I

Past history
Nil relevant

Antenatal period
Normal
Admitted at 40 weeks

21.00 hours
Spontaneous rupture of membranes – clear liquor draining
Contracting 1 in 5 minutes

Labour
Cervical os 2–3 cm dilated
Fetal scalp electrode applied
Intrauterine pressure catheter inserted

00.15 hours
Cervical os 3 cm dilated
Pethidine 100 mg and Sparine 25 mg given intramuscularly

03.10 hours
Cervical os 5 cm dilated

06.00 hours
Cervical os 7 cm dilated

08.45 hours
Epidural analgesia commenced

09.15 hours
CTG

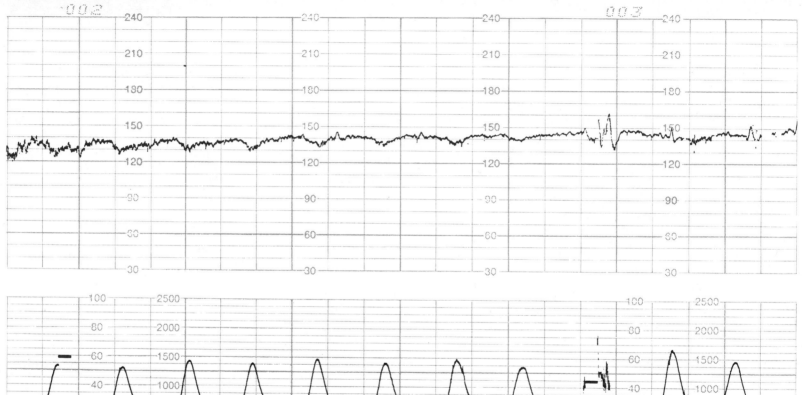

9500-8005/SON

CTG

1 What do you notice about the baseline?

2 What do you notice about the baseline variability?

3 What type of decelerations, if any, are present?

4 What do you notice about the uterine activity?

5 What is the most probable cause of fetal heart rate abnormality shown on this trace?

6 What treatment and/or intervention would you consider necessary for this fetal heart rate pattern?

NOTES

1

2

3

4

5

6

ANALYSIS

1 Baseline 130–135 b.p.m., rising during CTG

2 Variability less than 5 b.p.m., accelerations with some contractions

3 Shallow early decelerations

4 Contracting 5 in 10 minutes

5 Head compression
Variability reduced, previously normal, acceleration present – probably sleep phase

6 Change maternal position
If variability does not increase within 40 minutes, fetal blood sampling is indicated

OUTCOME

09.45 hours
Second stage of labour diagnosed
Variability now 5–10 b.p.m.

11.00 hours
Commenced pushing

12.02 hours
Spontaneous vertex delivery
Live girl
Apgar score 9/1 9/5
Birthweight 4.220 kg

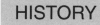
HISTORY

27-year-old gravida I, para 0

Past history
Nil relevant

Antenatal period
Normal
Admitted at 41 weeks with spontaneous
rupture of membranes – clear liquor draining;
contracting 1 in 5 minutes

Labour

12.45 hours
Cervical os 3 cm dilated
Fetal scalp electrode applied
Intrauterine pressure catheter inserted

14.30 hours
CTG

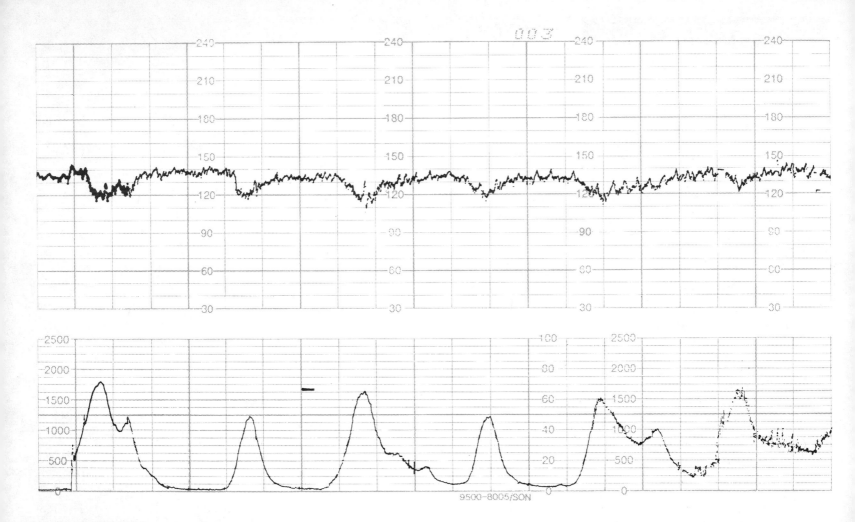

9500-8005/SON

CTG

1 What do you notice about the baseline?

2 What do you notice about the baseline variability?

3 What type of decelerations, if any, are present?

4 What do you notice about the uterine activity?

5 What is the most probable cause of fetal heart rate abnormality shown on this trace?

6 What treatment and/or intervention would you consider necessary for this fetal heart rate pattern?

NOTES

1

2

3

4

5

6

ANALYSIS

1 Baseline 130–135 b.p.m.

2 Variability 5–10 b.p.m.

3 Early decelerations

4 Contracting 1 in 3 minutes, varying in strength

5 Head compression

6 Change maternal position
  Observe for further abnormalities

OUTCOME

15.30 hours
Cervical os 5 cm dilated

16.30 hours
Second stage diagnosed
Commenced pushing
Deep variable decelerations noted

16.55 hours
Rotational forceps delivery
Live girl
Apgar score 6/1 9/5
Birthweight 2.630 kg
Cord around neck × 3

CASE STUDY

12

27-year-old gravida III, para 2

Past history
Nil relevant

Antenatal period
Urinary tract infection treated at 24 weeks'
gestation
Normal progress
Admitted at 41 weeks' gestation in
spontaneous labour

Labour

13.30 hours
Cervical os 5 cm dilated, membranes intact
Initial CTG normal

15.50 hours
CTG recommenced, external recordings

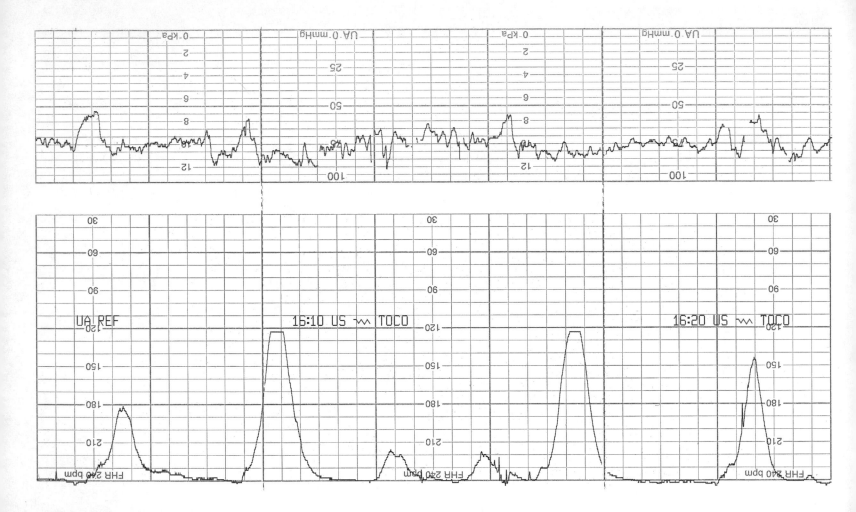

CTG

1 What do you notice about the baseline?

2 What do you notice about the baseline variability?

3 What type of decelerations, if any, are present?

4 What do you notice about the uterine activity?

5 What is the most probable cause of fetal heart rate abnormality shown on this trace?

6 What treatment and/or intervention would you consider necessary for this fetal heart rate pattern?

NOTES

1

2

3

4

5

6

ANALYSIS

1 Baseline, unable to interpret

2 Variability, probably within normal limits

3 No decelerations

4 Contracting 3 in 10 minutes, varying in strength

5 Probably normal CTG, paper has been loaded into machine upside down
Despite this the CTG is recorded as being satisfactory in the case notes·on two occasions

6 Change paper

OUTCOME

Paper rectified after 1 hour
Progressed to normal delivery 3 hours later
Live girl
Apgar score 9/1 9/5
Birthweight 3.380 kg

HISTORY

20-year-old gravida I, para 0

Past history
Nil relevant

Antenatal period
No problems
Admitted at 38 weeks with spontaneous
rupture of membranes and contractions

Labour

13.00 hours
Cervical os 3 cm dilated
Fetal scalp electrode applied
Intrauterine pressure catheter inserted

15.00 hours
No progress, Syntocinon infusion
commenced

16.30 hours
Epidural analgesia commenced

18.25 hours
Cervical os 6 cm dilated

19.30 hours
Syntocinon infusing at 10 mU/min
CTG

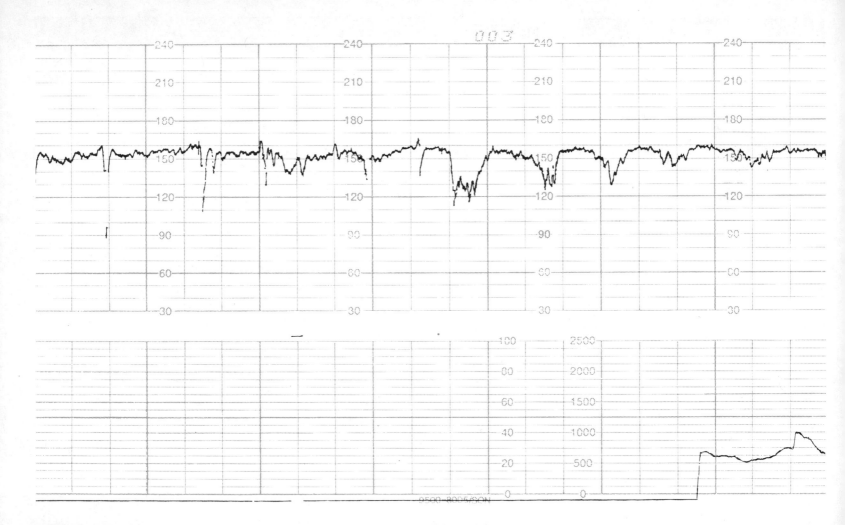

CTG

1 What do you notice about the baseline?

2 What do you notice about the baseline variability?

3 What type of decelerations, if any, are present?

4 What do you notice about the uterine activity?

5 What is the most probable cause of fetal heart rate abnormality shown on this chart?

6 What treatment and/or intervention would you consider necessary for this fetal heart rate pattern?

NOTES

1

2

3

4

5

6

ANALYSIS

1 Baseline 150–155 b.p.m.

2 Variability 5 b.p.m.

3 Decelerations cannot be classified as no contractions monitored

4 Contractions not monitored

5 No cause can be attributed

6 Monitor contractions
Classify decelerations and take appropriate action

OUTCOME

Contractions monitored, decelerations classified as early

20.55 hours
Second stage of labour diagnosed

22.00 hours
Commenced pushing

22.55 hours
Spontaneous vertex delivery
Live girl
Apgar score 9/1 9/5
Birthweight 2.780 kg

Late decelerations

14

HISTORY

21-year-old gravida I, para 0

Past history
Nil relevant

Antenatal period
Normal
Admitted at 41 weeks, contracting 1 in 5 minutes
Admission CTG – shallow late decelerations

Labour

06.05 hours
Cervical os 2 cm dilated
Artificial rupture of membranes – fresh meconium-stained liquor draining
Fetal scalp electrode applied
Contractions monitored externally

07.15 hours
CTG

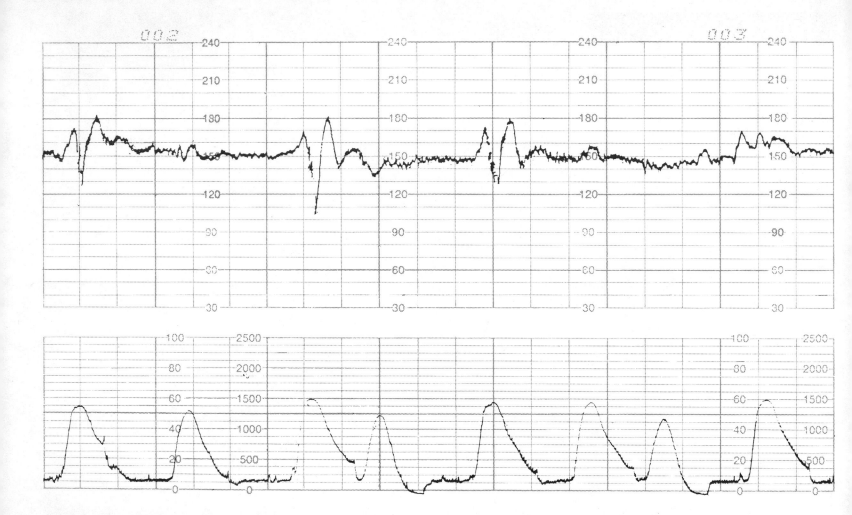

CTG

1 What do you notice about the baseline?

2 What do you notice about the baseline variability?

3 What type of decelerations, if any, are present?

4 What do you notice about the uterine activity?

5 What is the most probable cause of fetal heart rate abnormality shown on this trace?

6 What treatment and/or intervention would you consider necessary for this fetal heart rate pattern?

NOTES

1

2

3

4

5

6

ANALYSIS

1 Baseline 130–140 b.p.m.

2 Variability 5–10 b.p.m.

3 Late decelerations

4 Contracting 3 in 10 minutes

5 Fetal hypoxia
  Variability normal – suggests fetus not
  compromised

6 Change maternal position
  Give facial oxygen
  Commence intravenous infusion
  Fetal blood sampling is indicated

OUTCOME

08.15 hours
Cervical os 2 cm dilated
Fetal blood sampling performed: pH 7.18,
base excess –8
Caesarean section performed
Live boy
Apgar score 4/1 9/5
Birthweight 3.450 kg
Placenta appeared infarcted

15

HISTORY

23-year-old gravida II, para 1

Past history
Nil relevant

Antenatal period
Normal
Admitted at 39 weeks in spontaneous labour,
contracting 1 in 5 minutes
Admission CTG

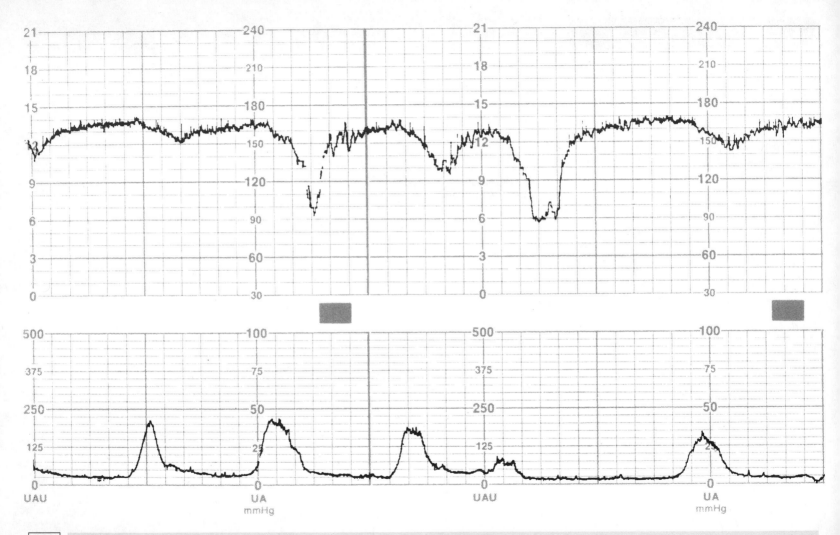

UAU   UA mmHg   UAU   UA mmHg

CTG	NOTES
1 What do you notice about the baseline?	1
2 What do you notice about the baseline variability?	
3 What type of decelerations, if any, are present?	2
	3
4 What do you notice about the uterine activity?	
5 What is the most probable cause of fetal heart rate abnormality shown on this trace?	4
6 What treatment and/or intervention would you consider necessary for this fetal heart rate pattern?	5
	6

ANALYSIS

1 Baseline 160–165 b.p.m.

2 Variability – external recording, therefore not accurate; appears less than 5 b.p.m.

3 Late decelerations

4 Irregular contractions, 2–3 in 10 minutes

5 Fetal hypoxia

6 Change maternal position
Give facial oxygen
Vaginal examination to assess cervical dilation
Commence intravenous fluids
If cervical os not dilated, consider induction of labour or caesarean section

OUTCOME

01.40 hours
Cervical os 5 cm dilated
Artificial rupture of membranes – fresh, thick meconium-stained liquor draining
Fetal scalp electrode applied
CTG – late decelerations continue

02.00 hours
Caesarean section performed
Live boy
Apgar score 2/1 10/5
Birthweight 2.88 kg
Placenta appears unhealthy

16

HISTORY

27-year-old gravida I, para 0

Past history
Nil relevant

Antenatal period
Normal
Admitted at 41 weeks with history of
diminished fetal movements for 3 days
Mild contractions for 2 hours
Admission CTG

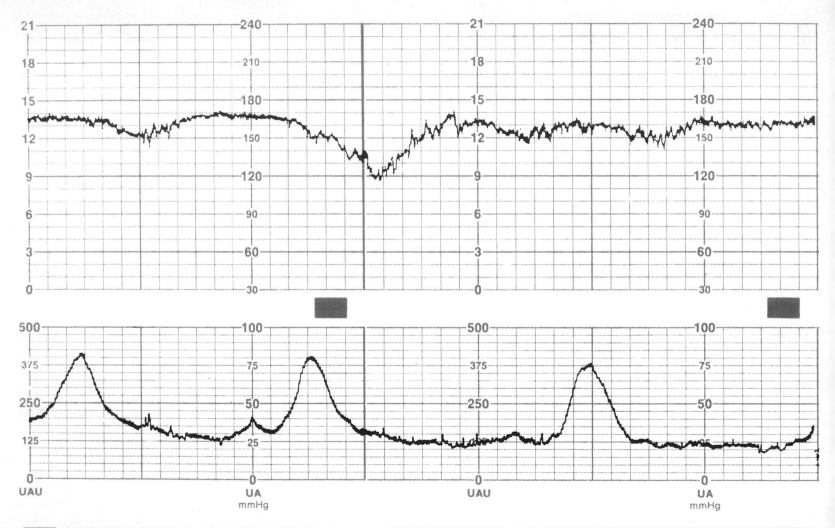

CTG	NOTES
1 What do you notice about the baseline?	1
2 What do you notice about the baseline variability?	
3 What type of decelerations, if any, are present?	2
4 What do you notice about the uterine activity?	3
5 What is the most probable cause of fetal heart rate abnormality shown on this trace?	4
6 What treatment and/or intervention would you consider necessary for this fetal heart rate pattern?	5
	6

ANALYSIS

1 Baseline 160–165 b.p.m.

2 Variability – externally monitored, therefore not accurate; appears reduced

3 Late decelerations

4 Contracting 1–2 in 10 minutes

5 Fetal hypoxia
   Note history of diminished fetal movements

6 Change maternal position
   Give facial oxygen
   Vaginal examination to assess cervical dilation
   If cervix favourable, artificial rupture of membranes to assess the colour of the liquor and to perform fetal blood sampling
   Prepare for delivery while these actions are performed
   If cervix not favourable, deliver

OUTCOME

24.00 hours
Cervical os 5 cm dilated
Artificial rupture of membranes – fresh meconium-stained liquor draining
Fetal scalp electrode applied – resulting CTG of poor quality
Fetal blood sampling performed: pH 7.09, base excess −10

01.48 hours
Caesarean section performed
Live boy
Apgar score 4/1 8/5
Birthweight 3.330 kg

HISTORY

22-year-old gravida II, para 0 + 1

Past history
Benign intracranial hypertension diagnosed 2 years ago

Antenatal period
Admitted at 34 weeks with raised blood pressure of 160/105 and proteinuria

36 weeks
Blood pressure rising, 170/115; proteinuria increasing
Ultrasound scan – reduced liquor volume

Labour

00.30 hours
Cervix 1 cm long, cervical os 1.5 cm dilated
Artificial rupture of membranes – clear liquor draining
Fetal scalp electrode applied
Intrauterine pressure catheter inserted
Syntocinon infusion commenced

01.25 hours
Epidural analgesia commenced

01.40 hours
Syntocinon infusing at 4 mU/min
CTG

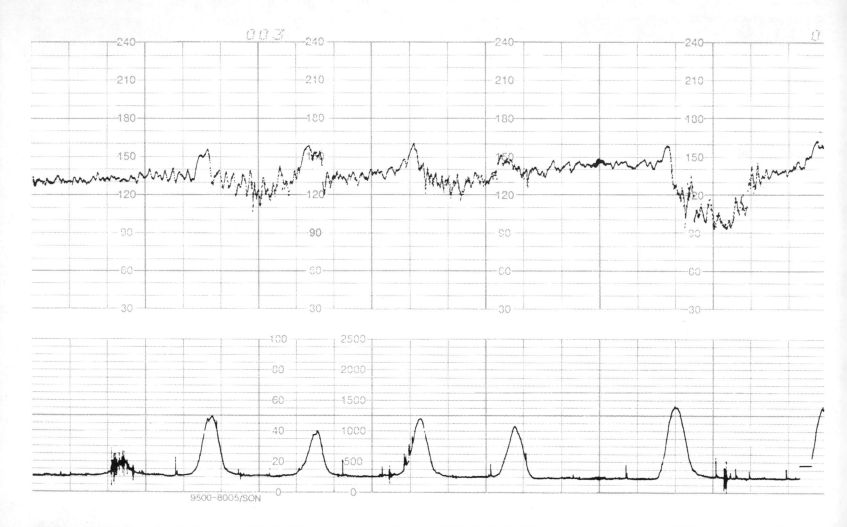

9500-8005/SON

CTG

1 What do you notice about the baseline?

2 What do you notice about the baseline variability?

3 What type of decelerations, if any, are present?

4 What do you notice about the uterine activity?

5 What is the most probable cause of fetal heart rate abnormality shown on this trace?

6 What treatment and/or intervention would you consider necessary for this fetal heart rate pattern?

NOTES

1

2

3

4

5

6

ANALYSIS

1 Baseline 135–145 b.p.m.

2 Variability 5–10 b.p.m.

3 Late decelerations

4 Contracting 3 in 10 minutes, varying in strength

5 Fetal hypoxia
  Note hypertension and reduced liquor volume

6 Change maternal position
  Give facial oxygen
  Stop Syntocinon infusion, increase intravenous infusion
  Fetal blood sampling is indicated
  Prepare for delivery

OUTCOME

03.10 hours
Cervical os 3 cm dilated
Syntocinon infusion stopped

04.30 hours
CTG – late decelerations continue
Fetal blood sampling attempted – failed

05.10 hours
Caesarean section performed
Live girl
Apgar score 9/1 9/5
Birthweight 2.360 kg
Thick meconium noted at delivery
Multiple placental infarcts

HISTORY

25-year-old gravida I, para 0

Past history
Nil relevant

Antenatal period
Normal
Admitted in spontaneous labour at 41 weeks, contracting 1 in 5 minutes

Labour

16.30 hours
Cervical os 2 cm dilated
Artificial rupture of membrane – clear liquor draining
Fetal scalp electrode applied
Contractions monitored externally

17.30 hours
CTG

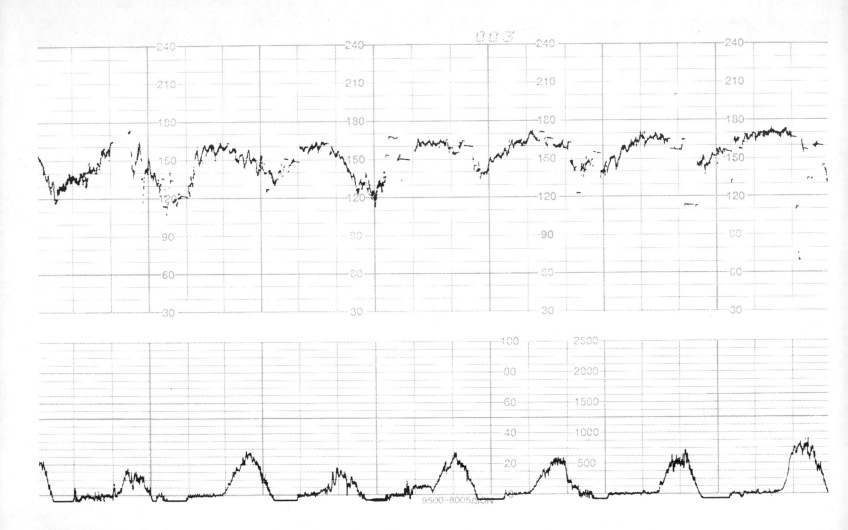

CTG	NOTES
1 What do you notice about the baseline?	1
2 What do you notice about the baseline variability?	
3 What type of decelerations, if any, are present?	2
4 What do you notice about the uterine activity?	3
5 What is the most probable cause of fetal heart rate abnormality shown on this trace?	4
6 What treatment and/or intervention would you consider necessary for this fetal heart rate pattern?	5
	6

ANALYSIS

1 Baseline 160–165 b.p.m.

2 Variability 5 b.p.m.

3 Late decelerations

4 Contracting 3 in 10 minutes, not
  adequately monitored

5 Fetal hypoxia

6 Change maternal position
  Give facial oxygen
  Commence intravenous infusion
  Fetal blood sampling is indicated
  As baseline tachycardia present with
  decreased variability, prepare for delivery
  while these actions are being performed

OUTCOME

18.00 hours
Fetal blood sampling performed: pH 7.32

18.30 hours
Meconium-stained liquor noted
Late decelerations now more prolonged

19.00 hours
Second stage of labour diagnosed

19.15 hours
Rotational forceps delivery
Live boy
Apgar score 8/1 9/5
Birthweight 3.700 kg
Large number of placental infarcts noted

HISTORY

37-year-old gravida V, para III + I

Past history
Insulin-dependent, diabetic for 6 years

Antenatal period
Amniocentesis at 17 weeks – indication, maternal age
Two admissions for control of diabetes

Labour
Surgical induction at 38 weeks

10.45 hours
Cervix 1.5 cm long, cervical os 1.5 cm dilated
Artificial rupture of membranes – clear liquor draining
Fetal scalp electrode applied
Intrauterine pressure catheter inserted
Syntocinon infusion commenced

14.50 hours
Cervical os 4 cm dilated

15.15 hours
Epidural analgesia commenced

16.50 hours
Syntocinon infusing at 8 mU/min.
Contractions now monitored externally
CTG

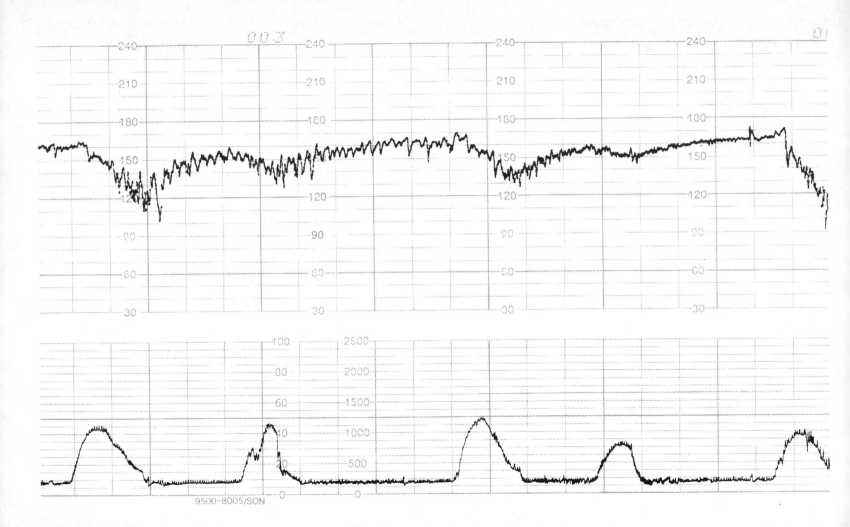

9500-8005/SON

CTG

1 What do you notice about the baseline?

2 What do you notice about the baseline variability?

3 What type of decelerations, if any, are present?

4 What do you notice about the uterine activity?

5 What is the most probable cause of fetal heart rate abnormality shown on this trace?

6 What treatment and/or intervention would you consider necessary for this fetal heart rate pattern?

NOTES

1

2

3

4

5

6

ANALYSIS

1 Baseline 150–160 b.p.m.

2 Variability appears reduced, possibly sinusoidal pattern in places

3 Late decelerations

4 Contractions 2–3 in 10 minutes, varying in strength

5 Fetal hypoxia
  Note maternal diabetes

6 Change maternal position
  Give facial oxygen
  Increase intravenous infusion
  Take sample of blood for glucose level
  Fetal blood sampling is indicated
  Prepare for delivery

OUTCOME

17.15 hours
Fetal blood sampling performed: pH 7.28, base excess –6
Blood glucose estimation 4 mmol/l
CTG – pattern continues

17.58 hours
Caesarean section performed
Live boy
Apgar score 9/1 9/5
Birthweight 3.500 kg

Variable decelerations

HISTORY

20-year-old gravida I, para 0

Past history
Nil relevant

Antenatal period
Normal
Admitted at 40 weeks with contractions for 3 minutes

Labour

05.30 hours
Cervical os 5 cm dilated
Artificial rupture of membranes – clear liquor draining
Fetal scalp electrode applied
Intrauterine pressure catheter inserted

06.45 hours
Pethidine 100 mg and Sparine 25 mg given intramuscularly

08.35 hours
Cervical os 6 cm dilated

10.15 hours
Epidural analgesia commenced

11.00 hours
Cervical os 9 cm dilated

12.30 hours
CTG

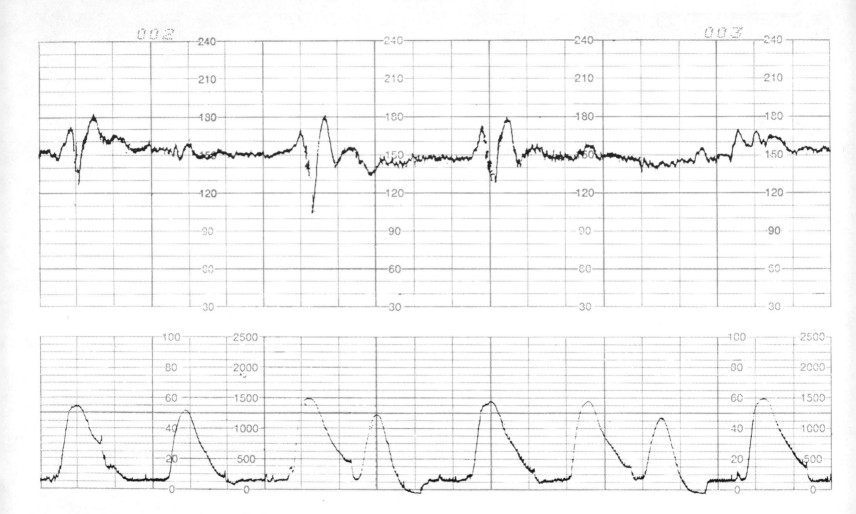

CTG

1 What do you notice about the baseline?

2 What do you notice about the baseline variability?

3 What type of decelerations, if any, are present?

4 What do you notice about the uterine activity?

5 What is the most probable cause of fetal heart rate abnormality shown on this trace?

6 What treatment and/or intervention would you consider necessary for this fetal heart rate pattern?

NOTES

1

2

3

4

5

6

ANALYSIS

1 Baseline 145–150 b.p.m.

2 Variability less than 5 b.p.m.

3 Variable decelerations

4 Contracting 4–5 in 10 minutes

5 Cord compression

6 Change maternal position
  Give facial oxygen
  Increase intravenous infusion
  Observe for further abnormalities
  If variability decreases any further, or if
  decelerations become more severe, fetal
  blood sampling is indicated

OUTCOME

13.00 hours
Second stage of labour diagnosed

13.30 hours
Commenced pushing

14.25 hours
No progress made
Straight forceps delivery
Live boy
Apgar score 9/1 9/5
Birthweight 3.250 kg
Cord around neck × 1

HISTORY

23-year-old gravida I, para 0

Past history
Nil relevant

Antenatal period
Normal
Admitted at $41\frac{1}{2}$ weeks for surgical induction of labour

Labour

15.15 hours
Cervix 1 cm long, cervical os 2 cm dilated
Artificial rupture of membranes – clear liquor draining
Fetal scalp electrode applied
Intrauterine pressure catheter inserted.
Syntocinon infusion commenced

17.40 hours
Pethidine 100 mg and Sparine 25 mg given intramuscularly

18.15 hours
Cervical os 8 cm dilated
Clear liquor draining

20.20 hours
Second stage of labour confirmed
Commenced pushing

21.00 hours
Vertex advancing
CTG

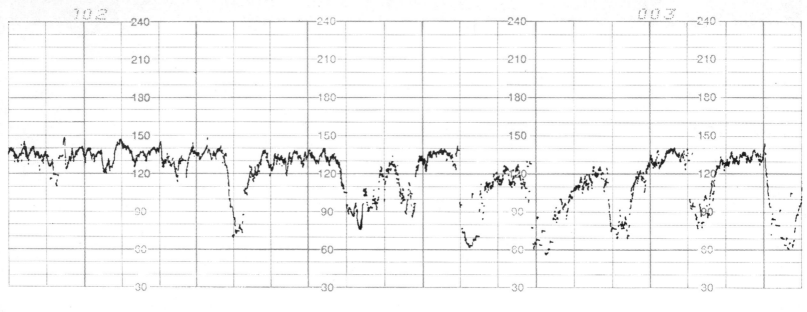
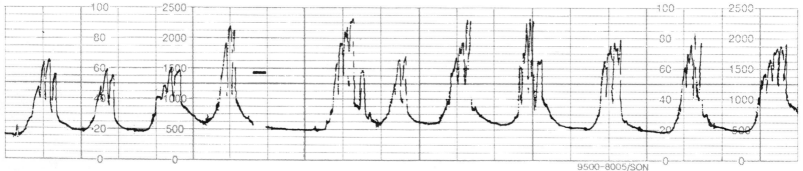

9500-8005/SON

CTG

1 What do you notice about the baseline?

2 What do you notice about the baseline variability?

3 What type of decelerations, if any, are present?

4 What do you notice about the uterine activity?

5 What is the most probable cause of fetal heart rate abnormality shown on this trace?

6 What treatment and/or intervention would you consider necessary for this fetal heart rate pattern?

NOTES

1

2

3

4

5

6

ANALYSIS

1 Baseline 130–140 b.p.m.

2 Variability 5–10 b.p.m.

3 Variable decelerations

4 Contracting 4–5 in 10 minutes

5 Cord compression

6 Change maternal position
  Give facial oxygen
  In view of normal variability and baseline,
  continue pushing

OUTCOME

21.57 hours
Spontaneous vertex delivery
Live boy
Apgar score 6/1 9/5
Birthweight 4.130 kg
Cord around neck × 1, tightly

HISTORY

25-year-old gravida I, para 0

Past history
Nil relevant

Antenatal period
Normal
Admitted at 41 weeks, contracting 1 in 5 minutes

Labour

10.30 hours
Cervical os 7 cm dilated
Artificial rupture of membranes – clear liquor draining
Fetal scalp electrode applied

12.50 hours
Cervical os 8 cm dilated
Epidural analgesia commenced

14.30 hours
CTG

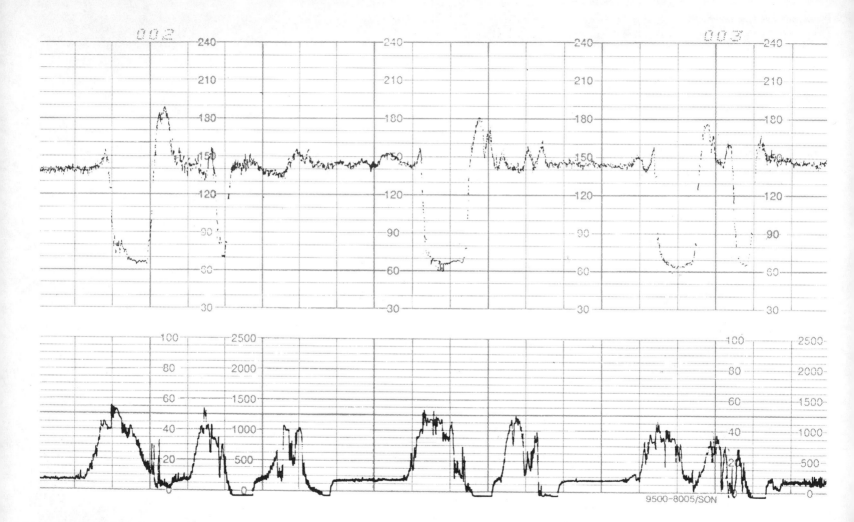

9500-8005/SON

CTG

1 What do you notice about the baseline?

2 What do you notice about the baseline variability?

3 What type of decelerations, if any, are present?

4 What do you notice about the uterine activity?

5 What is the most probable cause of fetal heart rate abnormality shown on this trace?

6 What treatment and/or intervention would you consider necessary for this fetal heart rate pattern?

NOTES

1

2

3

4

5

6

ANALYSIS

1 Baseline 140–145 b.p.m.

2 Variability 5 b.p.m., some accelerations

3 Variable decelerations

4 Contracting 3 in 10 minutes, varying in strength

5 Cord compression

6 Change maternal position
  Give facial oxygen
  Vaginal examination to assess cervical dilation and exclude cord prolapse
  Fetal blood sampling is indicated

OUTCOME

14.45 hours
Second stage of labour diagnosed
Fetal blood sampling performed: pH 7.29, base excess –6

15.05 hours
Commenced pushing

15.30 hours
No improvement in CTG

15.42 hours
Straight forceps delivery
Live girl
Apgar score 3/1 8/5
Birthweight 3.060 kg
Cord around neck × 1

HISTORY

28-year-old gravida I, para 0

Past history
Nil relevant

Antenatal period
Normal
Admitted at 41 weeks, contracting 1 in 5 minutes, spontaneous rupture of membranes

Labour

03.30 hours
Cervical os 4 cm dilated
Clear liquor draining
Fetal scalp electrode applied
Contractions monitored externally

04.00 hours
Epidural analgesia commenced

05.30 hours
Second stage diagnosed

06.30 hours
Commenced pushing

07.00 hours
No progress being made
CTG

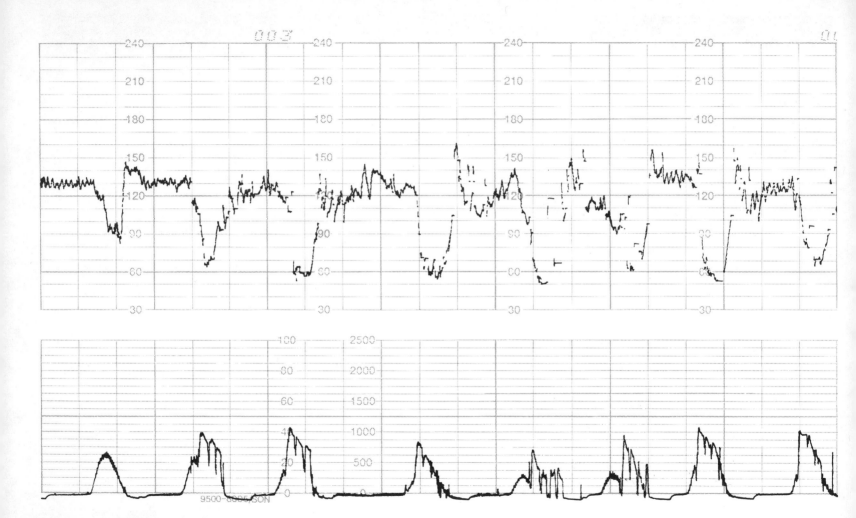

CTG	NOTES
1 What do you notice about the baseline?	1
2 What do you notice about the baseline variability?	
3 What type of decelerations, if any, are present?	2
4 What do you notice about the uterine activity?	3
5 What is the most probable cause of fetal heart rate abnormality shown on this trace?	4
6 What treatment and/or intervention would you consider necessary for this fetal heart rate pattern?	5
	6

ANALYSIS

1 Baseline 125–130 b.p.m.

2 Variability 5–10 b.p.m.

3 Variable decelerations

4 Contracting 3–4 in 10 minutes

5 Cord compression

6 Change maternal position
  Give facial oxygen
  Increase intravenous infusion
  In view of little progress being made,
  prepare for delivery

OUTCOME

07.40 hours
Straight forceps delivery
Live girl
Apgar score 9/1 9/5
Birthweight 2.840 kg
Cord around neck × 1

24

HISTORY

27-year-old gravida I, para 0

Past history
Nil relevant

Antenatal period
Subchorionic bleed noted at 29 weeks on ultrasound scan
Follow-up scans normal
Pregnancy progressed well
Admitted at term plus 11 days for surgical induction of labour

Labour

10.00 hours
Artificial rupture of membranes – clear liquor draining
Initial external CTG normal

10.45 hours
Syntocinon infusion commenced
Continuous external CTG commenced

16.30 hours
Epidural analgesia in progress
CTG normal

01.15 hours
Cervical os 7 cm dilated, clear liquor draining
Progress in labour slow

01.50 hours
CTG

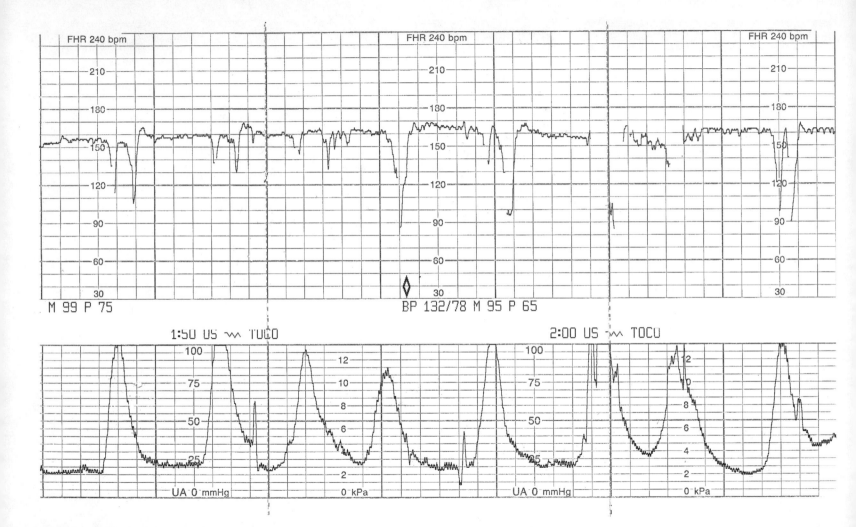

FHR 240 bpm

FHR 240 bpm

FHR 240 bpm

M 99 P 75

BP 132/78 M 95 P 65

1:50 US ∿ TOCO

2:00 US ∿ TOCO

UA 0 mmHg

0 kPa

UA 0 mmHg

0 kPa

CTG

1 What do you notice about the baseline?

2 What do you notice about the baseline variability?

3 What type of decelerations, if any, are present?

4 What do you notice about the uterine activity?

5 What is the most probable cause of fetal heart rate abnormality shown on this trace?

6 What treatment and/or intervention would you consider necessary for this fetal heart rate pattern?

NOTES

1

2

3

4

5

6

ANALYSIS

1 Baseline 155–160 b.p.m.

2 Variability less than 5, no accelerations

3 Variable decelerations

4 Contracting 3–4 in 10 minutes

5 Cord compression
Baseline slightly raised although has
remained constant throughout labour

6 Change maternal position
Record maternal temperature and pulse
rate
Fetal blood sampling may be indicated if
pattern persists

OUTCOME

Mother apyrexial, pulse rate 92 b.p.m.
Variable decelerations reduce, occasional
decelerations only

05.00 hours
Progressed to second stage of labour

06.50 hours
No progress made with maternal effort
Cephalic presentation still one-fifth palpable
abdominally
Occasional variable decelerations continue
Emergency caesarean section performed
Live boy
Apgar score 9/1 9/5
Birthweight 3.840 kg
Cord gases: pH 7.40, base excess −3.2

25

HISTORY

14-year-old gravida I, para 0

Past history
Nil relevant

Antenatal period
Normal
Admitted at 38 weeks with contractions

Labour

20.00 hours
Cervical os 3–4 cm dilated
Artificial rupture of membranes – clear liquor draining
Fetal scalp electrode applied
Intrauterine pressure catheter inserted

20.30 hours
CTG

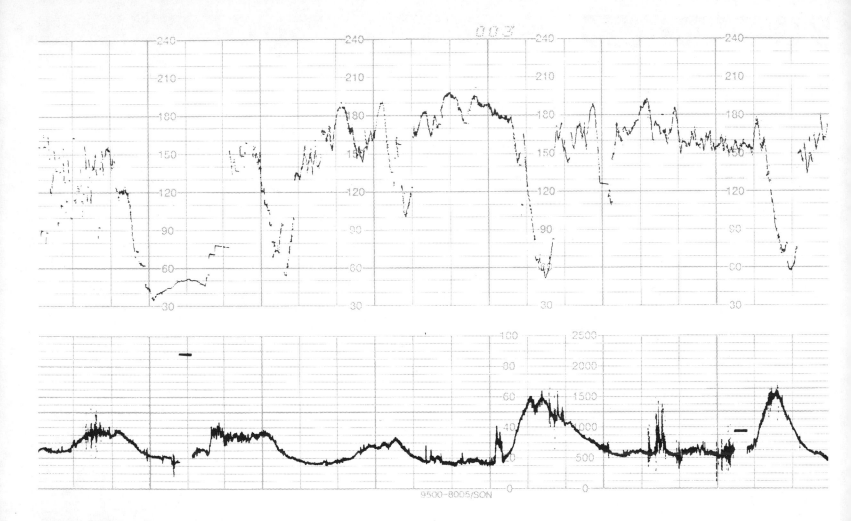

CTG	NOTES
1 What do you notice about the baseline?	1
2 What do you notice about the baseline variability?	
3 What type of decelerations, if any, are present?	2
4 What do you notice about the uterine activity?	3
5 What is the most probable cause of fetal heart rate abnormality shown on this trace?	
6 What treatment and/or intervention would you consider necessary for this fetal heart rate pattern?	4
	5
	6

ANALYSIS

1 Baseline 155 b.p.m.

2 Variability 5–15 b.p.m.

3 Variable decelerations

4 Contractions not monitored adequately, appear 3 in 10 minutes

5 Cord compression, resulting in fetal hypoxia

6 Change maternal position
  Give facial oxygen
  Fetal blood sampling is indicated
  Prepare for delivery
  Vaginal examination to exclude cord prolapse

OUTCOME

Variable decelerations continue

21.20 hours
Caesarean section performed
Live girl
Apgar score 9/1 9/5
Birthweight 2.710 kg
No cord around neck

26

HISTORY

32-year-old gravida II, para 2

Past history
Caesarean section 3 years ago for twin
pregnancy

Antenatal period
Normal
Admitted at 42 weeks with spontaneous
rupture of membranes and contractions

Labour

23.55 hours
Cervical os 2 cm dilated – clear liquor
draining
Fetal scalp electrode applied
Contractions monitored externally

00.10 hours
Pethidine 100 mg and Sparine 25 mg given
intramuscularly

02.15 hours
Cervical os 4 cm dilated
Intrauterine pressure catheter inserted

03.00 hours
CTG

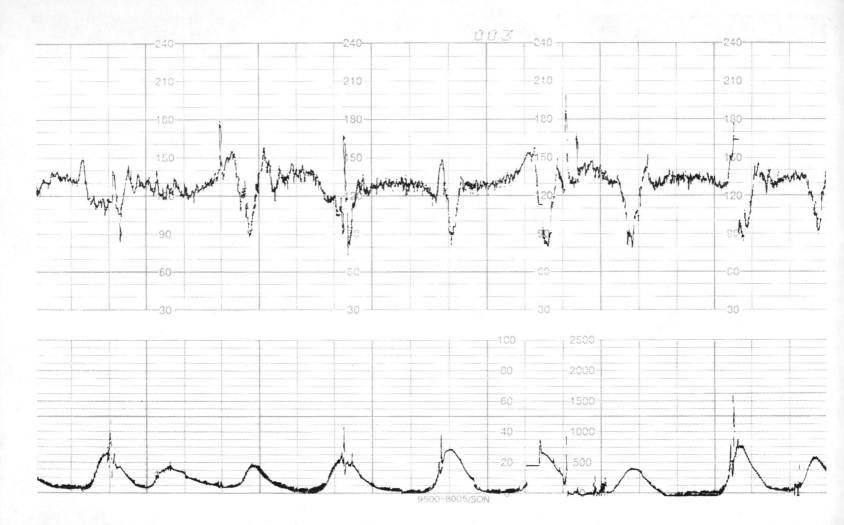

9500-8005/SON

CTG	NOTES
1 What do you notice about the baseline?	1
2 What do you notice about the baseline variability?	
3 What type of decelerations, if any, are present?	2
4 What do you notice about the uterine activity?	3
5 What is the most probable cause of fetal heart rate abnormality shown on this trace?	4
6 What treatment and/or intervention would you consider necessary for this fetal heart rate pattern?	5
	6

ANALYSIS

1 Baseline 125–135 b.p.m.

2 Variability 5–10 b.p.m.

3 Variable decelerations

4 Contracting 4 in 10 minutes

5 Cord compression

6 Change maternal position
Give facial oxygen
Increase intravenous infusion
Observe for further abnormalities
If pattern persists, fetal blood sampling is
indicated

OUTCOME

04.00 hours
Cervical os 9 cm dilated
Loop of cord in front of head
Transferred to theatre; second stage of
labour diagnosed on arrival

04.17 hours
Straight forceps delivery
Live boy
Apgar score 8/1 9/5
Birthweight 3.380 kg

CASE STUDY

27

HISTORY

30-year-old gravida I, para 0

Past history
Nil relevant

Antenatal period
Normal
Admitted at 40 weeks with contractions for 2 hours
Early decelerations noted on admission CTG

Labour

22.00 hours
Cervical os 3 cm dilated
Artificial rupture of membranes – clear liquor draining
Fetal scalp electrode applied
Intrauterine pressure catheter inserted

22.30 hours
Epidural analgesia commenced

24.00 hours
Variable decelerations noted
Cervical os 7 cm dilated

01.25 hours
Second stage diagnosed
Commenced pushing

02.00 hours
CTG

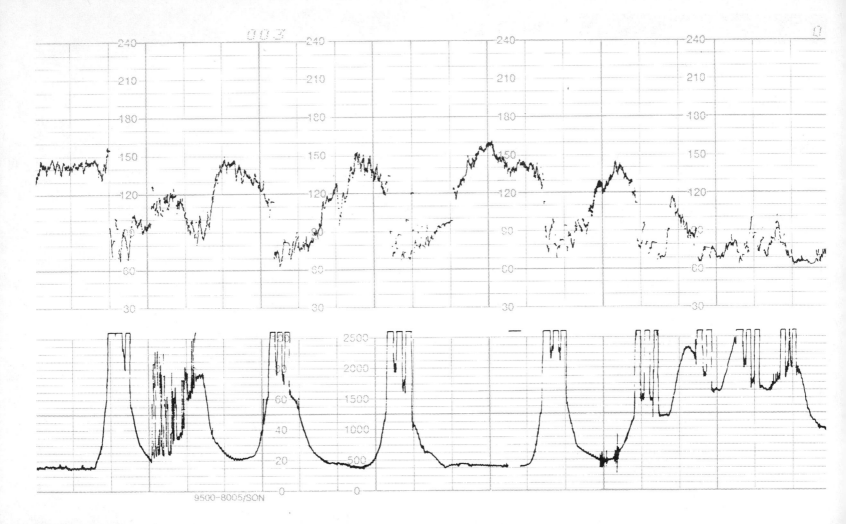

9500–8005/SON

CTG	NOTES
1 What do you notice about the baseline?	1
2 What do you notice about the baseline variability?	
3 What type of decelerations, if any, are present?	2
4 What do you notice about the uterine activity?	3
5 What is the most probable cause of fetal heart rate abnormality shown on this trace?	4
6 What treatment and/or intervention would you consider necessary for this fetal heart rate pattern?	
	5
	6

ANALYSIS

1 Baseline 145–150 b.p.m.

2 Variability 5–10 b.p.m.

3 Variable decelerations followed by prolonged deceleration

4 Contracting 3–4 in 10 minutes, varying in strength

5 Variable decelerations followed by prolonged deceleration – cord occlusion

6 Change maternal position
   Give facial oxygen
   Increase intravenous fluids
   Prepare for delivery

OUTCOME

02.26 hours
Straight forceps delivery
Live boy
Apgar score 9/1 9/5
Birthweight 3.100 kg
Cord around neck × 2 tightly

Reduced variability

HISTORY

25-year-old gravida I, para 0

Past history
Nil relevant

Antenatal period
Normal
Admitted at 40 weeks with contractions

Labour

19.30 hours
Cervical os 3 cm dilated
Artificial rupture of membranes – clear liquor draining
Fetal scalp electrode applied
Contractions monitored externally
CTG reactive

20.20 hours
Pethidine 100 mg and Sparine 25 mg given intramuscularly

20.40 hours
CTG

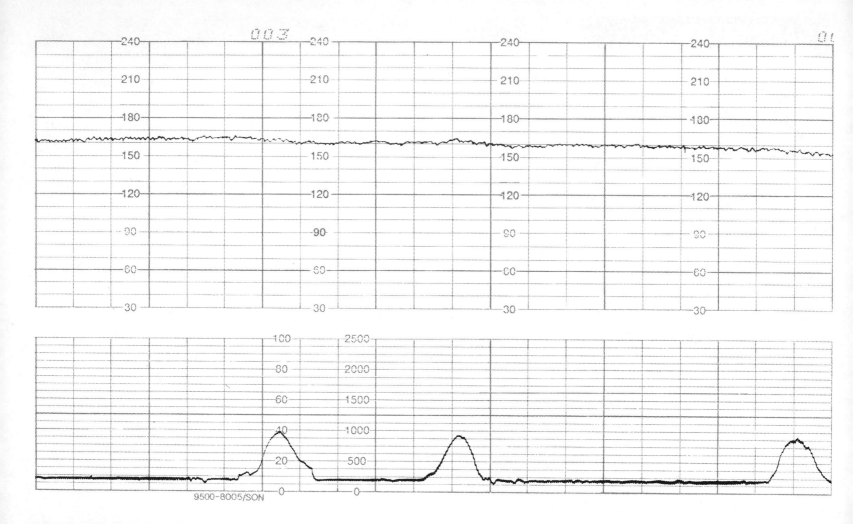

9500-8005/SON

CTG

1 What do you notice about the baseline?

2 What do you notice about the baseline variability?

3 What type of decelerations, if any, are present?

4 What do you notice about the uterine activity?

5 What is the most probable cause of fetal heart rate abnormality shown on this trace?

6 What treatment and/or intervention would you consider necessary for this fetal heart rate pattern?

NOTES

1

2

3

4

5

6

ANALYSIS

1 Baseline 160 b.p.m.

2 Variability little or none present

3 No decelerations

4 Contractions irregular, 1–2 in 10 minutes

5 In view of reactive CTG prior to analgesia, probably pethidine induced

6 Observe for further abnormalities
If pattern persists for longer than 40 minutes, fetal blood sampling is indicated

OUTCOME

02.00 hours
Cervical os 6 cm dilated
CTG now reactive

07.30 hours
Second stage of labour diagnosed

08.20 hours
Spontaneous vertex delivery
Live girl
Apgar score 7/1 9/5
Birthweight 4.040 kg

HISTORY

21-year-old gravida I, para 0

Past history
Nil relevant

Antenatal period
Normal
Admitted at 41 weeks with contractions

Labour

08.00 hours
Cervical os 4 cm dilated
Artificial rupture of membranes – clear liquor draining
Fetal scalp electrode applied
Intrauterine pressure catheter inserted
CTG reactive

08.30 hours
Pethidine 100 mg and Sparine 25 mg given intramuscularly

08.50 hours
CTG

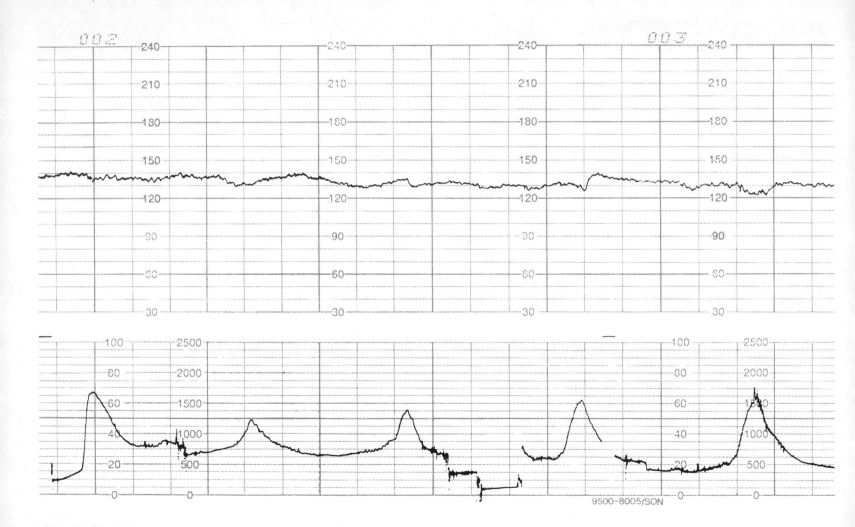

9500-8005/SON

CTG

1 What do you notice about the baseline?

2 What do you notice about the baseline variability?

3 What type of decelerations, if any, are present?

4 What do you notice about the uterine activity?

5 What is the most probable cause of fetal heart rate abnormality shown on this trace?

6 What treatment and/or intervention would you consider necessary for this fetal heart rate pattern?

NOTES

1

2

3

4

5

6

ANALYSIS

1 Baseline 135 b.p.m.

2 Variability 1–2 b.p.m

3 No decelerations

4 Contracting 2–3 in 10 minutes

5 In view of reactive CTG prior to analgesia, pethidine induced

6 Observe for further abnormalities
   If pattern persists for longer than 40 minutes, fetal blood sampling is indicated

OUTCOME

09.15 hours
Variability returns to normal

11.30 hours
Cervical os 7 cm dilated

11.50 hours
Epidural analgesia commenced

14.30 hours
Second stage of labour diagnosed

15.30 hours
Commenced pushing

16.45 hours
Straight forceps delivery for delay in second stage
Live boy
Apgar score 9/1 9/5
Birthweight 4.040 kg

HISTORY

26-year-old gravida II, para 1

Past history
Nil relevant

Antenatal period
Normal
Admitted at 40 weeks, contracting 1 in 5 minutes

Labour

05.30 hours
Cervical os 1 cm dilated
Admission CTG normal
Allowed to mobilise

09.30 hours
Cervix thick, cervical os 2 cm dilated
Requesting epidural analgesia
Artificial rupture of membranes – clear liquor draining
Fetal scalp electrode applied
Contractions monitored externally

10.25 hours
Epidural analgesia commenced
Occasional mild variable decelerations noted on CTG

13.10 hours
Cervical os 3.5 cm dilated
Liquor clear
CTG

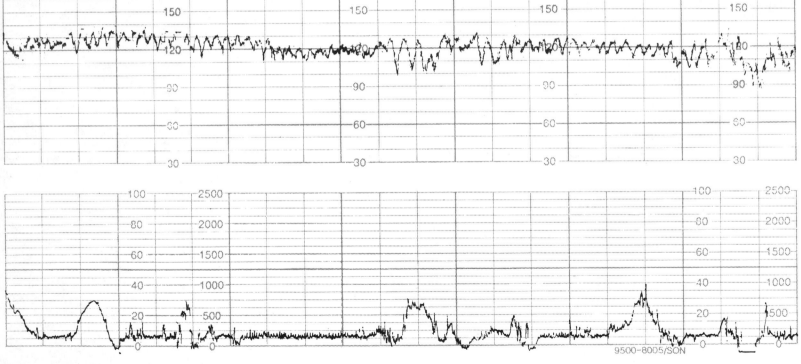

CTG

1 What do you notice about the baseline?

2 What do you notice about the baseline variability?

3 What type of decelerations, if any, are present?

4 What do you notice about the uterine activity?

5 What is the most probable cause of fetal heart rate abnormality shown on this trace?

6 What treatment and/or intervention would you consider necessary for this fetal heart rate pattern?

NOTES

1

2

3

4

5

6

ANALYSIS

1 Baseline 125–135 b.p.m.

2 Variability virtually absent; sinusoidal pattern

3 No decelerations

4 Contractions irregular, not monitored adequately

5 Preceding variable decelerations – cord occlusion probable, resulting in fetal hypoxia

6 Change maternal posture
  Give facial oxygen
  Increase intravenous fluids
  Fetal blood sampling is indicated
  Prepare for delivery

OUTCOME

14.00 hours
Variable decelerations occur again
Sinusoidal pattern remains

14.25 hours
Fetal blood sampling performed: pH 7.23, base excess −14.3

15.12 hours
Emergency caesarean section performed
Live boy
Apgar score 5/1 9/5
Birthweight 3.620 kg
Umbilical cord wrapped around body

HISTORY

32-year-old gravida IV, para 2 + 1

Past history
Previous mid-trimester abortion

Antenatal period
Normal progress
Admitted in spontaneous labour at 39 weeks' gestation

Labour

17.00 hours
Cervical os 5 cm dilated, membranes intact

17.58 hours
Pethidine 100 mg and Sparine 25 mg given intramuscularly

18.00 hours
CTG

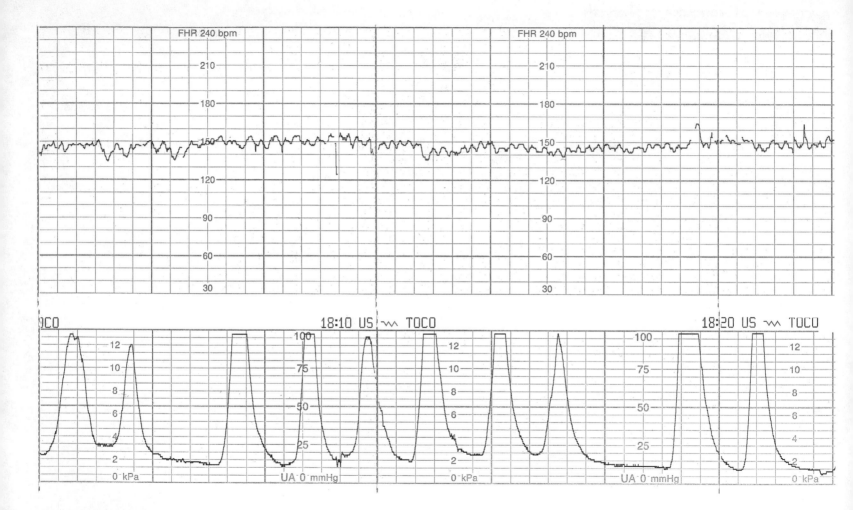

CTG	NOTES
1 What do you notice about the baseline?	1
2 What do you notice about the baseline variability?	
3 What type of decelerations, if any, are present?	2
4 What do you notice about the uterine activity?	3
5 What is the most probable cause of fetal heart rate abnormality shown on this trace?	4
6 What treatment and/or intervention would you consider necessary for this fetal heart rate pattern?	
	5
	6

ANALYSIS

1 Baseline 145–150 b.p.m.

2 Variability –? sinusoidal pattern initially, reverts to normal variability towards end of portion of CTG with small accelerations

3 No decelerations

4 Contracting 4 in 10 minutes

5 In view of normal variability previously, return to normal at end of CTG and absence of other abnormalities, probably pethidine induced

6 Continue to monitor the fetal heart
If pattern persists, consider artificial rupture of the membranes to assess the colour of the liquor

OUTCOME

Progressed rapidly to normal delivery at 19.00 hours
Live boy
Apgar score 9/1 9/5
Birthweight 2.96 kg

32

25-year-old gravida II, para 0 + 1

Past history
Deep venous thrombosis 4 years ago

Antenatal history
Treated with prophylactic subcutaneous heparin from 16 weeks
Admitted at 40 weeks, contracting 1 in 5 minutes

Labour

16.45 hours
Cervical os 2–3 cm dilated
Artificial rupture of membranes – fresh, thick meconium-stained liquor draining
Fetal scalp electrode applied
Contractions monitored externally
CTG

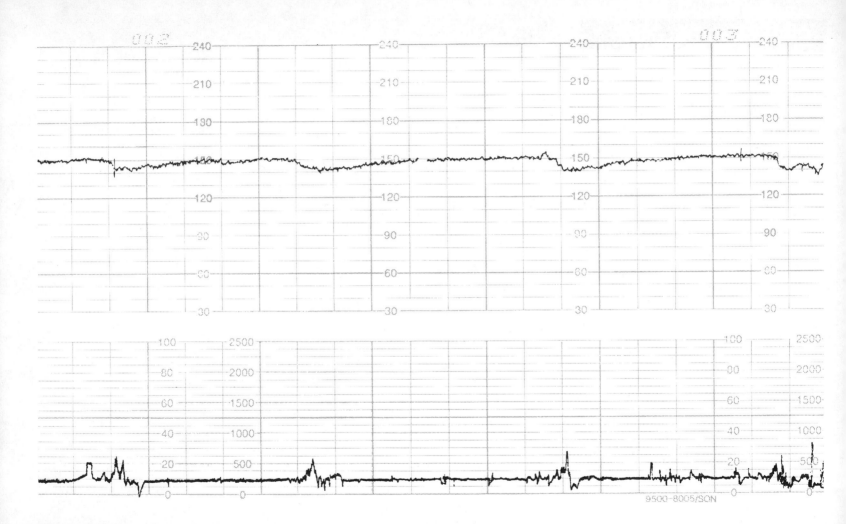

9500-8005/SON

CTG

1 What do you notice about the baseline?

2 What do you notice about the baseline variability?

3 What type of decelerations, if any, are present?

4 What do you notice about the uterine activity?

5 What is the most probable cause of fetal heart rate abnormality shown on this trace?

6 What treatment and/or intervention would you consider necessary for this fetal heart rate pattern?

NOTES

1

2

3

4

5

6

ANALYSIS	OUTCOME

ANALYSIS

1 Baseline 145–150 b.p.m.

2 Variability little or absent

3 Shallow decelerations, cannot be classified as contractions as not monitored adequately

4 Contractions not monitored adequately

5 Decreased variability, decelerations, presence of fresh meconium – fetal hypoxia

6 Change maternal position
Give facial oxygen
Prepare for delivery

OUTCOME

17.30 hours
Caesarean section performed
Live boy
Apgar score 8/1 10/5
Birthweight 3.100 kg

HISTORY

30-year-old gravida V, para III + 1

Past history
Firot baby unoxplainod otillbirth, at torm
All babies small for dates

Antenatal period

26 weeks
Growth scan performed – measurements on
10th centile

28 weeks
Repeat scan – growth now below 10th centile
Admitted at 33 weeks with diminished fetal
movements
Ultrasound scan – breech presentation,
growth below 10th centile, liquor volume
reduced for gestation
Admission CTG

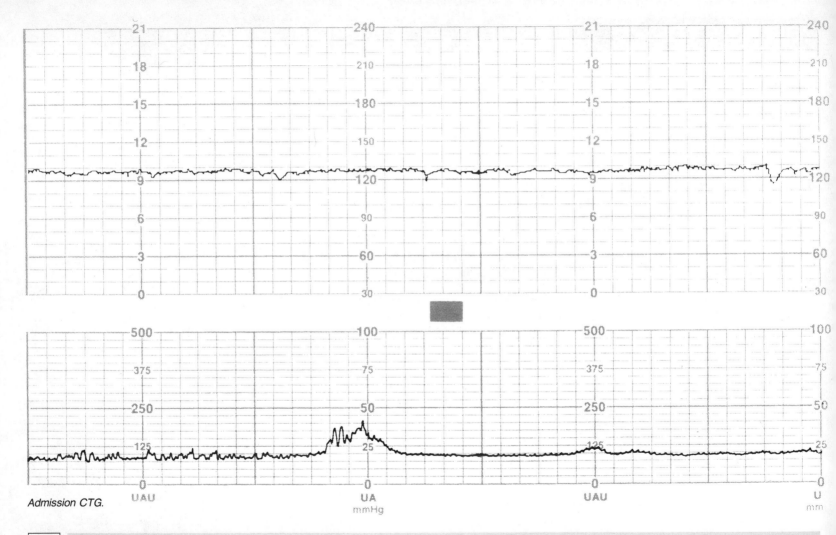

Admission CTG.

CTG

1 What do you notice about the baseline?

2 What do you notice about the baseline variability?

3 What type of decelerations, if any, are present?

4 What do you notice about the uterine activity?

5 What is the most probable cause of fetal heart rate abnormality shown on this trace?

6 What treatment and/or intervention would you consider necessary for this fetal heart rate pattern?

NOTES

1

2

3

4

5

6

ANALYSIS

1 Baseline 125 b.p.m.

2 Variability – external recording, therefore not accurate; appears to be little or absent

3 No decelerations

4 No contractions, one mild tightening only

5 In view of poor obstetric history, intrauterine growth retardation and diminished fetal movements, fetal hypoxia must be considered

6 Continue CTG; if pattern persists for longer than 40 minutes, consider delivery

OUTCOME

CTG discontinued; repeated following day

CASE STUDY

33

PART 2

OUTCOME [CONTINUED]

Following day CTG.

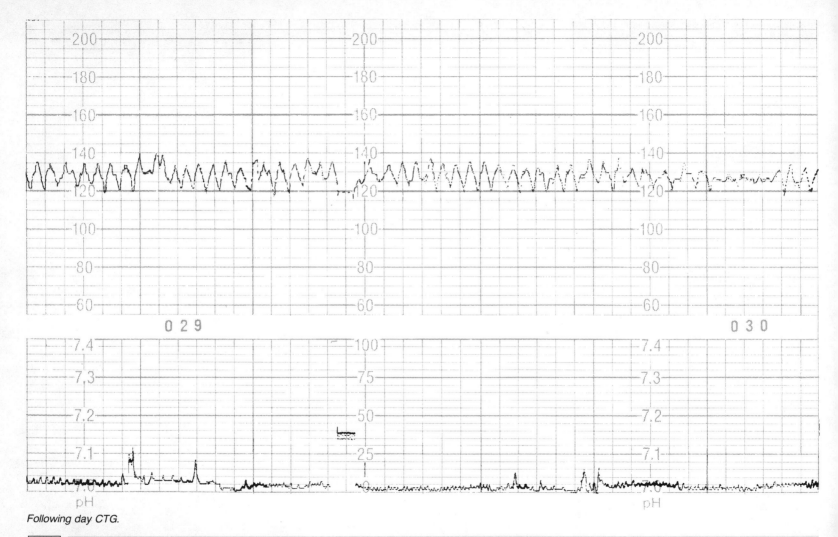

029

030

Following day CTG.

CTG	NOTES
1 What do you notice about the baseline?	1
2 What do you notice about the baseline variability?	
3 What type of decelerations, if any, are present?	2
4 What do you notice about the uterine activity?	3
5 What is the most probable cause of fetal heart rate abnormality shown on this trace?	4
6 What treatment and/or intervention would you consider necessary for this fetal heart rate pattern?	5
	6

ANALYSIS

1 Baseline difficult to determine, either 125 or 135 b.p.m.

2 Variability – external, therefore not accurate; appears to be absent, sinusoidal pattern

3 No decelerations

4 No contractions

5 In view of history (as before) and previous CTG – fetal hypoxia

6 Prepare for delivery

OUTCOME

CTG discontinued
Following day, no fetal heart heard
4 days later, vaginal breech delivery of stillborn baby
Birthweight 1.460 kg
Cord around neck × 3
Post-mortem report confirms intrauterine anoxia

Bradycardia

HISTORY

24-year-old gravida II, para I

Past history
Nil relevant

Antenatal period
Normal
Admitted at 41 weeks with contractions for 2 hours

Labour

05.20 hours
Cervical os 2 cm dilated
Fetal scalp electrode applied
Intrauterine pressure catheter inserted

05.40 hours
Epidural analgesia commenced

08.45 hours
Cervical os 6 cm dilated
CTG

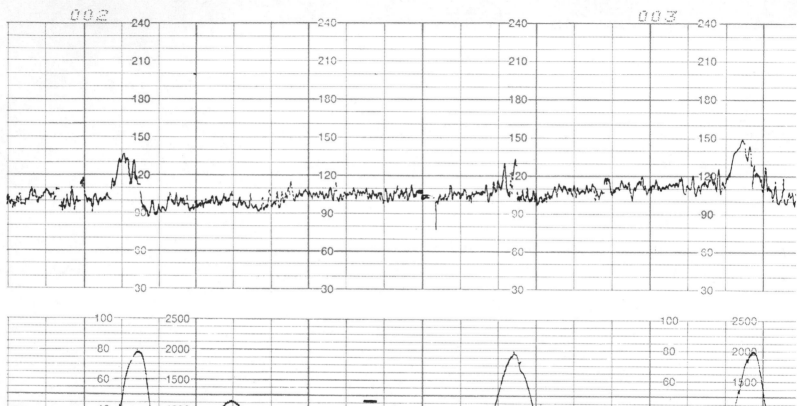

9500-8005/SON

CTG

1 What do you notice about the baseline?

2 What do you notice about the baseline variability?

3 What type of decelerations, if any, are present?

4 What do you notice about the uterine activity?

5 What is the most probable cause of fetal heart rate abnormality shown on this trace?

6 What treatment and/or intervention would you consider necessary for this fetal heart rate pattern?

NOTES

1

2

3

4

5

6

LIVERPOOL
JOHN MOORES UNIVERSITY
AVRIL ROBARTS LRC
TEL. 0151 231 4022

ANALYSIS

1 Baseline 100–110 b.p.m.

2 Variability 5–15 b.p.m.

3 No decelerations, some accelerations

4 Contracting 2 in 10 minutes, varying in strength

5 Low baseline, normal variability and accelerations – normal CTG

6 No action necessary
   Observe for further abnormalities

OUTCOME

14.00 hours
Progressed to second stage of labour

16.30 hours
Straight forceps delivery for delay in second stage
Live girl
Apgar score 10/1 10/5
Birthweight 4.250 kg

HISTORY

23-year-old gravida I, para 0

Past history
Nil relevant

Antenatal period
Normal
Admitted at 41 weeks with contractions

Labour

07.00 hours
Cervical os 3 cm dilated
Artificial rupture of membranes – clear liquor draining
Fetal scalp electrode applied
Contractions monitored externally

08.15 hours
CTG

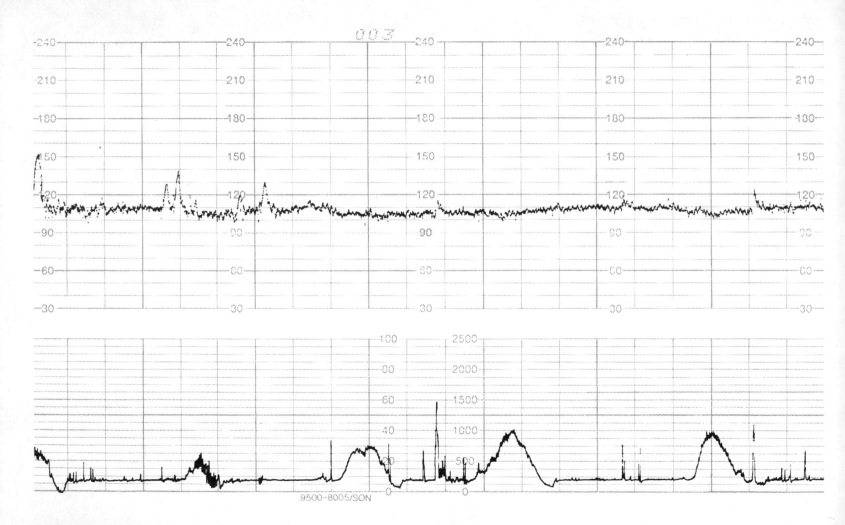

9500-8005/SON

CTG	NOTES
1 What do you notice about the baseline?	1
2 What do you notice about the baseline variability?	
3 What type of decelerations, if any, are present?	2
4 What do you notice about the uterine activity?	3
5 What is the most probable cause of fetal heart rate abnormality shown on this trace?	4
6 What treatment and/or intervention would you consider necessary for this fetal heart rate pattern?	
	5
	6

ANALYSIS

1 Baseline 100–110 b.p.m.

2 Variability less than 5 b.p.m.

3 No decelerations, some accelerations

4 Contracting 2 in 10 minutes, varying in strength

5 Low baseline variability reduced, although some accelerations are occurring
Normal CTG

6 If variability does not return to within normal limits, fetal blood sampling should be considered

OUTCOME

10.00 hours
Cervical os 5 cm dilated
CTG unchanged
Fetal blood sampling attempted – failed
Decision made to deliver
Caesarean section performed
Live boy
Apgar score 9/1 9/5
Birthweight 3.650 kg

Tachycardia

HISTORY

25-year-old gravida I, para 0

Past history
Nil relevant

Antenatal period
Normal
Admitted at 40 weeks, contracting 1 in 5 minutes for 2 hours

Labour

19.30 hours
Cervical os 3 cm dilated
Artificial rupture of membranes – clear liquor draining
Fetal scalp electrode applied
Contractions monitored externally

22.30 hours
Cervical os 5 cm dilated

22.45 hours
Epidural analgesia commenced

02.30 hours
Cervical os 6 cm dilated
CTG reactive, baseline 140 b.p.m.

05.30 hours
Cervical os 8 cm dilated

08.30 hours
Cervical os 9.5 cm dilated
Clear liquor draining
Maternal temperature 37.2°C

09.45 hours
Second stage of labour diagnosed

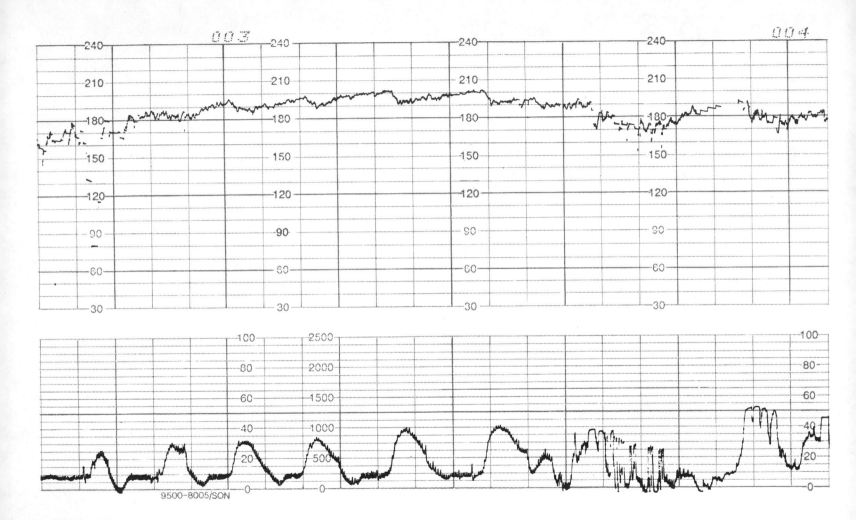

003

004

9500-8005/SON

CTG

1 What do you notice about the baseline?

2 What do you notice about the baseline variability?

3 What type of decelerations, if any, are present?

4 What do you notice about the uterine activity?

5 What is the most probable cause of fetal heart rate abnormality shown on this trace?

6 What treatment and/or intervention would you consider necessary for this fetal heart rate pattern?

NOTES

1

2

3

4

5

6

ANALYSIS

1 Baseline 190–200 b.p.m.

2 Variability less than 5 b.p.m.

3 No decelerations

4 Contracting 4 in 10 minutes, varying in
  strength

5 Maternal pyrexia could be responsible for
  fetal tachycardia
  Diminished variability – fetal hypoxia could
  be indicated

6 Change maternal position
  Reassess maternal temperature
  If pyrexia is evident, infection must be
  considered and appropriate treatment
  initiated
  Fetal blood sampling is contraindicated in
  view of maternal pyrexia
  Delivery should be expedited

OUTCOME

10.00 hours
Commenced pushing
CTG unchanged

10.30 hours
No progress
Straight forceps delivery
Live girl
Apgar score 7/1 9/5
Birthweight 3.460 kg

37

PART 1

HISTORY

19-year-old gravida I, para 0

Past history
Nil relevant

Antenatal period
Normal
Admitted at 40 weeks with spontaneous rupture of membranes and contractions

Labour

09.00 hours
Cervical os 3 cm dilated
Clear liquor draining
Fetal scalp electrode applied
Intrauterine pressure catheter inserted

09.20 hours
Epidural analgesia commenced

13.30 hours
Cervical os 4–5 cm dilated
Variable decelerations noted, baseline 125 b.p.m.
Fetal blood sampling performed: pH 7.32, base excess −2
Syntocinon infusion commenced

17.00 hours
Cervical os 8 cm dilated
Liquor clear
Maternal temperature 38.8°C
Syntocinon infusing at 18 mU/min

18.15 hours
CTG

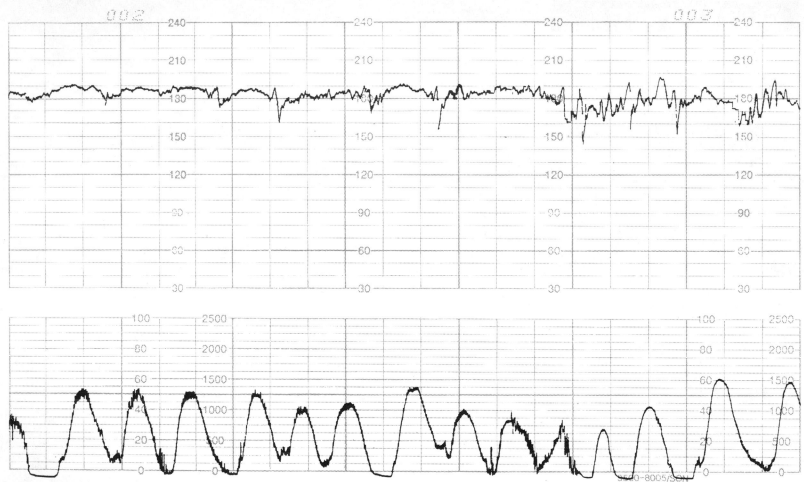

CTG at 18.15 hours.

CTG	NOTES
1 What do you notice about the baseline?	1
2 What do you notice about the baseline variability?	
3 What type of decelerations, if any, are present?	2
4 What do you notice about the uterine activity?	3
5 What is the most probable cause of fetal heart rate abnormality shown on this trace?	4
6 What treatment and/or intervention would you consider necessary for this fetal heart rate pattern?	
	5
	6

ANALYSIS

1 Baseline 180–190 b.p.m.

2 Variability 5–10 b.p.m.

3 No decelerations

4 Contracting 8 in 10 minutes

5 Variability normal, no decelerations, uncomplicated tachycardia – maternal pyrexia probable

6 Syntocinon infusion should be decreased in view of uterine hyperactivity
Observe for further abnormalities

OUTCOME

Labour continued

19.00 hours
Cervical os 8 cm dilated
Liquor discoloured:
? pus
? meconium

20.30 hours
Cervical os 8 cm dilated
Cephalic presentation; three-fifths palpable above pelvic brim
Syntocinon infusing at 10 mU/min
CTG – see Part 2, page 210.

OUTCOME [CONTINUED]

20.30 hours
CTG

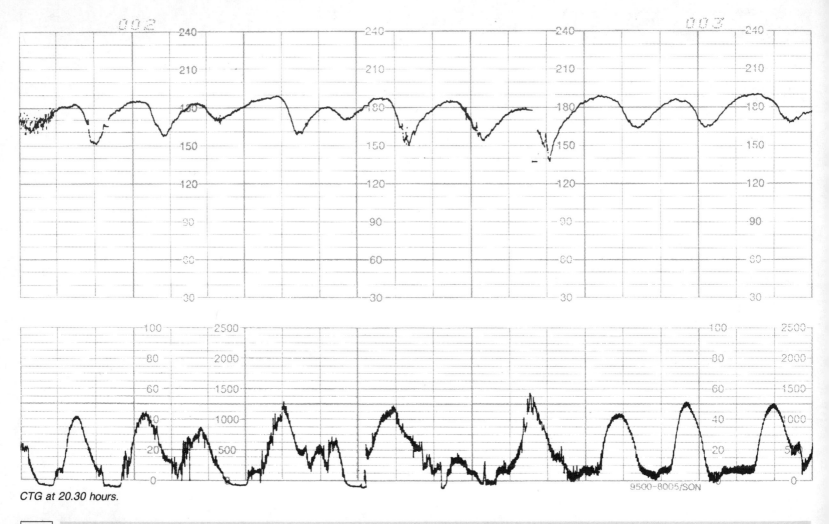

CTG at 20.30 hours.

CTG

1 What do you notice about the baseline?

2 What do you notice about the baseline variability?

3 What type of decelerations, if any, are present?

4 What do you notice about the uterine activity?

5 What is the most probable cause of fetal heart rate abnormality shown on this trace?

6 What treatment and/or intervention would you consider necessary for this fetal heart rate pattern?

NOTES

1

2

3

4

5

6

ANALYSIS

1 Baseline 180–190 b.p.m.

2 Variability virtually absent

3 Late decelerations

4 Contracting 4 in 10 minutes

5 Fetal tachycardia, late decelerations, loss of variability – fetal hypoxia

6 Change maternal position
  Give facial oxygen
  Increase intravenous fluids
  Prepare for delivery

OUTCOME

21.55 hours
Caesarean section performed
Live boy
Apgar score 1/1 9/5
Birthweight 4.200 kg
Cord around neck × 2, tightly
Fresh, thick meconium noted at delivery
Placenta appears very gritty and unhealthy

Complex

HISTORY

34-year-old gravida III, para 0 + 1

Past history
Two previous first trimester abortions

Antenatal period
Normal progress
Admitted at 42 weeks' gestation for surgical induction of labour

Labour

11.00 hours
Artificial rupture of membranes – clear liquor draining
Syntocinon infusion commenced
Fetal heart and contractions monitored externally

16.00 hours
Cervical os 4 cm dilated
Clear liquor draining
CTG normal, baseline 140 b.p.m.

17.30 hours
Epidural analgesia commenced

19.00 hours
Cervical os 8 cm dilated
CTG normal

21.00 hours
Second stage of labour diagnosed
Maternal temperature 37.6°C, pulse 100 b.p.m.
CTG

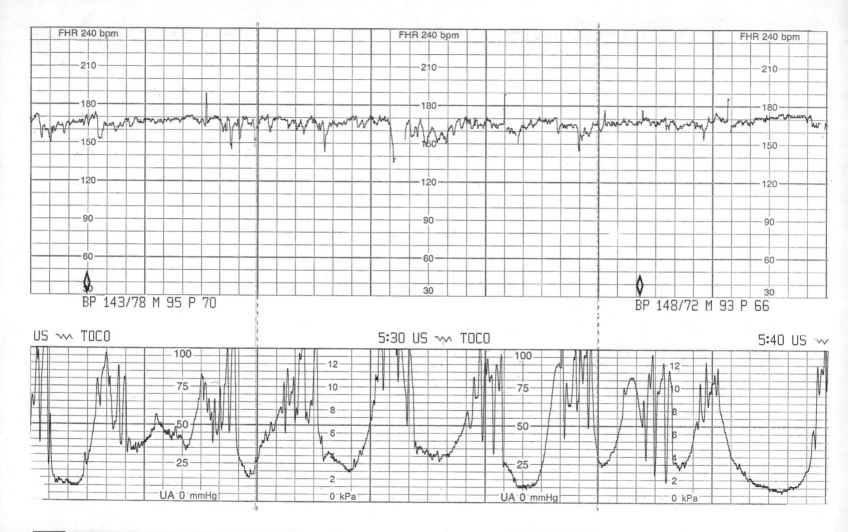

FHR 240 bpm
FHR 240 bpm
FHR 240 bpm

210
180
150
120
90
60
30

BP 143/78 M 95 P 70
BP 148/72 M 93 P 66

US ∿ TOCO
5:30 US ∿ TOCO
5:40 US ∿

100
75
50
25
UA 0 mmHg

12
10
8
6
2
0 kPa

CTG

1 What do you notice about the baseline?

2 What do you notice about the baseline variability?

3 What type of decelerations, if any, are present?

4 What do you notice about the uterine activity?

5 What is the most probable cause of fetal heart rate abnormality shown on this trace?

6 What treatment and/or intervention would you consider necessary for this fetal heart rate pattern?

NOTES

1

2

3

4

5

6

ANALYSIS

1 Baseline 165–170 b.p.m.

2 Variability 5–10, no accelerations

3 No decelerations

4 Contracting 3–4 in 10 minutes

5 Maternal pyrexia

6 Monitor mother's temperature and pulse, record on CTG
Consider taking blood cultures and treat with antibiotics

OUTCOME

21.30 hours
Commenced pushing

22.15 hours
No progress being made, prepared for instrumental delivery

22.40 hours
Straight forceps delivery
Live boy
Apgar score 5/1 9/5
Birthweight 3.50 kg
Cord gases: pH 7.33, base excess −10.7
Baby's temperature 37.2°C; ear, nose and cord swabs obtained, no growth

CASE STUDY

39

HISTORY

29-year-old gravida I, para 0

Past history
Nil relevant

Antenatal period
Admitted at 39 weeks, history of diminished fetal movements for 3 days
Admission CTG

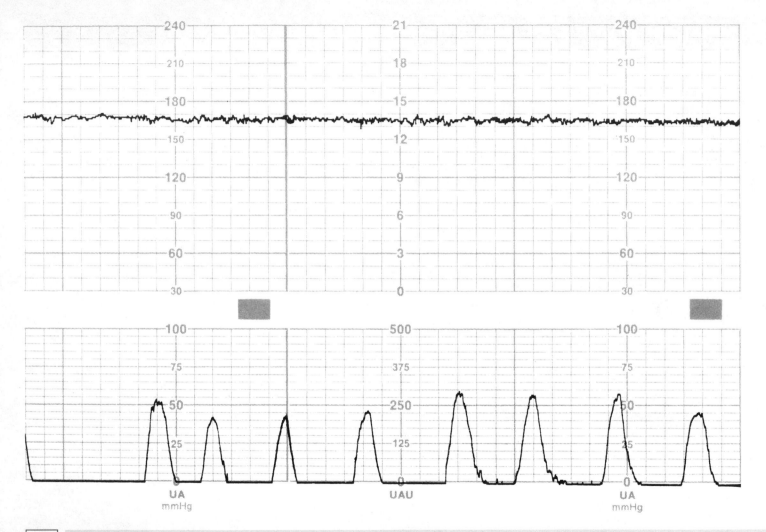

UA
mmHg

UAU

UA
mmHg

CTG

1 What do you notice about the baseline?

2 What do you notice about the baseline variability?

3 What type of decelerations, if any, are present?

4 What do you notice about the uterine activity?

5 What is the most probable cause of fetal heart rate abnormality shown on this trace?

6 What treatment and/or intervention would you consider necessary for this fetal heart rate pattern?

NOTES

1

2

3

4

5

6

ANALYSIS

1 Baseline 165 b.p.m.

2 Variability – external recording, therefore not accurate; appears virtually absent

3 No decelerations

4 Tightening 4–5 in 10 minutes, not painful

5 In view of history of diminished fetal movements, fetal hypoxia probable

6 Change maternal position
Give facial oxygen
Vaginal examination to assess cervical dilation, with a view to performing artificial rupture of membranes to observe colour of the liquor
Prepare for delivery

OUTCOME

Cervix posterior, 1 cm long, os 0.5 cm dilated
Caesarean section performed
Live girl
Apgar score 1/1 5/5
Birthweight 2.980 kg
Thick, fresh meconium noted at delivery
Baby transferred to neonatal unit
Listeriosis diagnosed at 2 days old; subsequently recovered

HISTORY

28-year-old gravida I, para 0

Past history
Nil rolovant

Antenatal period
Mild hypertension from 36 weeks
No proteinurea
Prostin induction of labour at 39 weeks' gestation

Labour

04.00 hours
Cervical os 4 cm dilated
Artificial rupture of membranes performed – clear liquor draining
Epidural analgesia commenced
Continuous external fetal monitoring in progress

05.10 hours
CTG

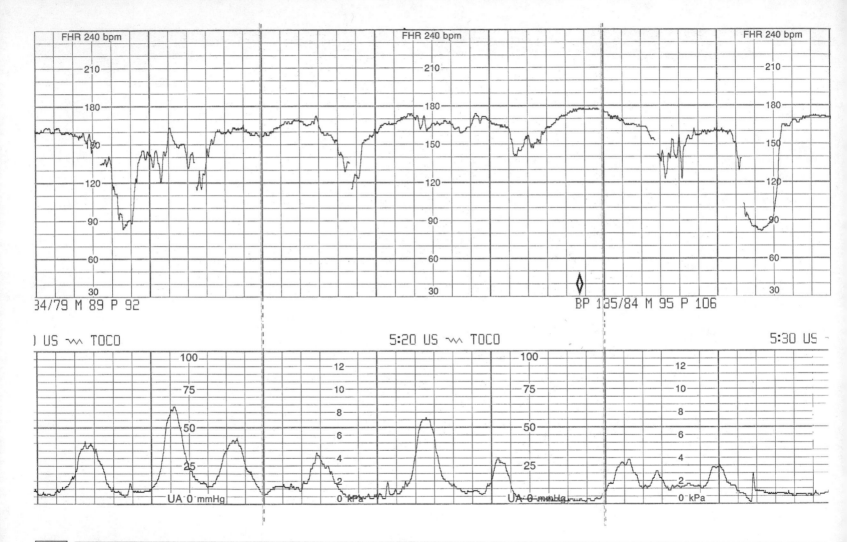

FHR 240 bpm

210
180
150
120
90
60
30

34/79 M 89 P 92

FHR 240 bpm

210
180
150
120
90
60
30

BP 135/84 M 95 P 106

FHR 240 bpm

210
180
150
120
90
60
30

US ᜼ TOCO

5:20 US ᜼ TOCO

5:30 US

100
75
50
25
UA 0 mmHg

12
10
8
6
4
2
0 kPa

100
75
50
25
UA 0 mmHg

12
10
8
6
4
2
0 kPa

CTG

1 What do you notice about the baseline?

2 What do you notice about the baseline variability?

3 What type of decelerations, if any, are present?

4 What do you notice about the uterine activity?

5 What is the most probable cause of fetal heart rate abnormality shown on this trace?

6 What treatment and/or intervention would you consider necessary for this fetal heart rate pattern?

NOTES

1

2

3

4

5

6

ANALYSIS

1 Baseline initially 160 b.p.m. rising to 180 b.p.m.

2 Variability less than 5, no accelerations

3 Variable decelerations

4 Contracting 3–4 in 10 minutes, irregular in strength and frequency

5 Cord compression
   Fetal tachycardia may be due to maternal pyrexia, although in view of increasing baseline and reduction in variability, fetal hypoxia should be excluded

6 Record maternal temperature
   Change maternal position
   Administer facial oxygen
   Discontinue any oxytocic infusion
   Consider fetal blood sampling

OUTCOME

Maternal temperature 37.5°C
Variable decelerations persist, with tachycardia, variability improves

06.10 hours
Fetal blood sampling performed: pH 7.34, base excess −3.6

09.00 hours
Cervical os 8–9 cm dilated

09.30 hours
Maternal temperature now 36.8°C
CTG as before
Repeat fetal blood sampling performed: pH 7.37, base excess −3.1

10.15 hours
Cervical os 8 cm dilated, therefore decision made for emergency caesarean section
Live girl
Apgar score 7/1 9/5
Birthweight 3.320 kg
Cord gases: pH 7.34, base excess −2.7

41

HISTORY

30-year-old gravida I, para 0

Past history
Nil relovant

Antenatal period
Admitted at 31 weeks with pregnancy-induced hypertension
Admission CTG normal
Blood pressure stabilised

32 weeks
Ultrasound scan shows good growth and normal liquor volume
Routine CTG 2 days later

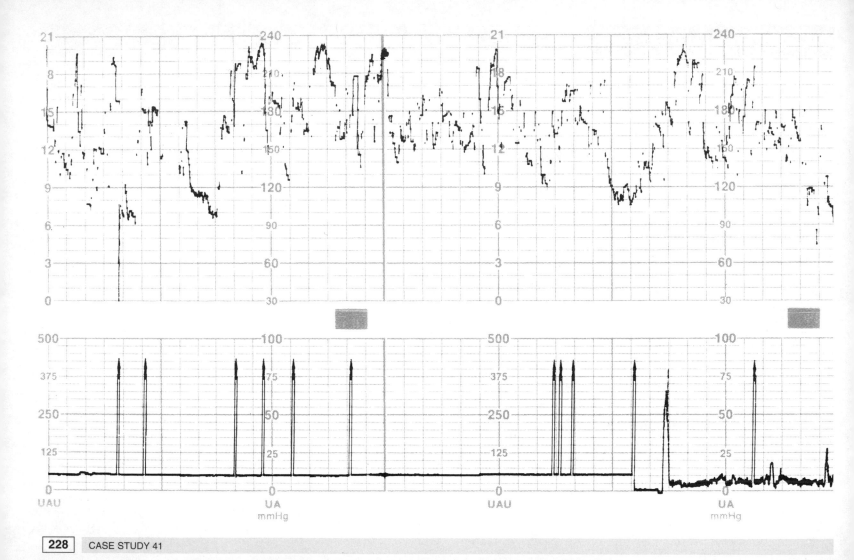

CTG	NOTES
1 What do you notice about the baseline?	1
2 What do you notice about the baseline variability?	
3 What type of decelerations, if any, are present?	2
4 What do you notice about the uterine activity?	3
5 What is the most probable cause of fetal heart rate abnormality shown on this trace?	4
6 What treatment and/or intervention would you consider necessary for this fetal heart rate pattern?	5
	6

ANALYSIS

Impossible to interpret this CTG

6 Fetal heart sounded irregular
   Repeat CTG – similar pattern

OUTCOME

Ultrasound scan performed
Structurally normal heart – atrial flutter
diagnosed
Cardiology opinion sought
Mother digitalised
Following day – ultrasound scan shows fetal
heart in normal sinus rhythm
CTG repeated 2 days later – see following
trace

35 weeks
Blood pressure unstable
Caesarean section performed
Live girl
Apgar score 4/1 9/5
Birthweight 1.810 kg
Baby discharged at 3 weeks old – no
problems

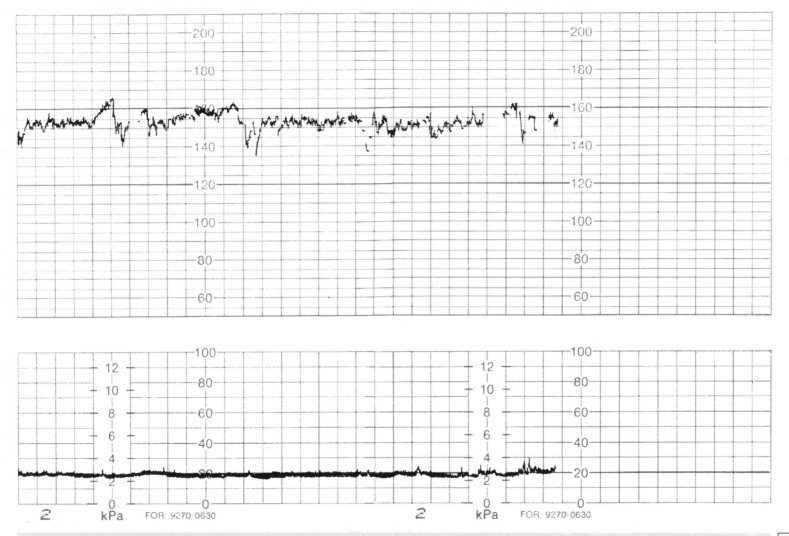

FOR: 9270-0630

FOR: 9270-0630

HISTORY

26-year-old gravida II, para 0 + 1

Past history
Nil relevant

Antenatal period
Normal
Admitted at 41 weeks for surgical induction of labour

Labour

12.30 hours
Cervix 0.5 cm long, cervical os 2 cm dilated
Artificial rupture of membranes – clear liquor draining
Fetal scalp electrode applied
Intrauterine pressure catheter inserted

13.45 hours
Epidural analgesia commenced

15.00 hours
Cervix unchanged from 12.30 hours
Syntocinon infusion commenced

17.00 hours
Cervical os 3–4 cm dilated

19.15 hours
Cervical os 9 cm dilated

21.15 hours
Cervical os 9 cm dilated
Syntocinon infusing at 8 mU/min
CTG

9500-8005/SON

CTG

1 What do you notice about the baseline?

2 What do you notice about the baseline variability?

3 What type of decelerations, if any, are present?

4 What do you notice about the uterine activity?

5 What is the most probable cause of fetal heart rate abnormality shown on this trace?

6 What treatment and/or intervention would you consider necessary for this fetal heart rate pattern?

NOTES

1

2

3

4

5

6

ANALYSIS

1 Baseline 140–145 b.p.m.

2 Variability less than 5 b.p.m.

3 Some decelerations initially, cannot be classified as no contractions monitored

4 Contractions not monitored adequately

5 CTG normal to this point
Decreased variability could be due to fetal sleep; cause for decelerations cannot be identified until they are classified

6 Change maternal position
Give facial oxygen
If pattern continues for 40 minutes or longer, fetal blood sampling is indicated

OUTCOME

00.30 hours
Second stage of labour diagnosed
Umbilical cord in vagina
Transferred to theatre
Rotational forceps delivery attempted – failed
Caesarean section performed
Live boy
Apgar score 9/1 9/5
Birthweight 4.100 kg

HISTORY

27-year-old gravida IV, para 0 + III

Past history
Three spontaneous mid-trimester abortions

Antenatal period

16 weeks
Cervical cerclage

37 weeks
Cervical suture removed
Admitted at 38 weeks with contractions, since
14.00 hours

Labour

15.00 hours
Cervical os 9.5 cm dilated
Artificial rupture of membranes – clear liquor
draining
Fetal scalp electrode applied
Contractions not monitored
CTG

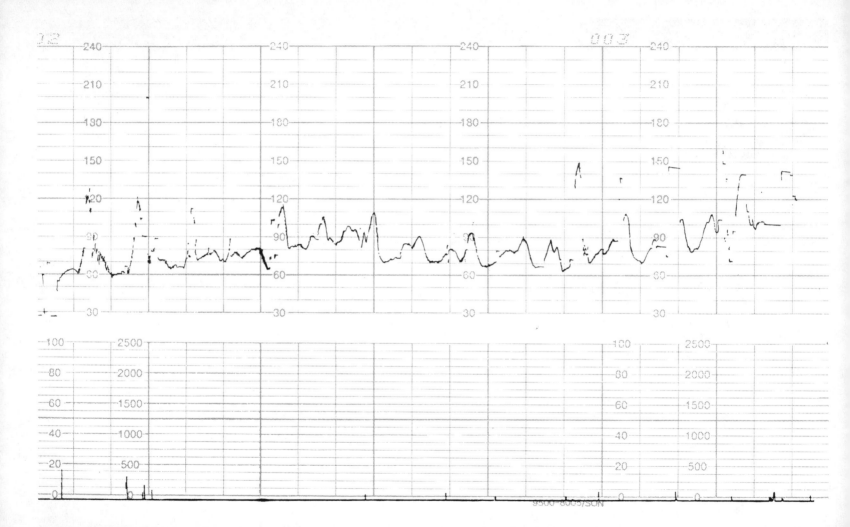

CTG

1 What do you notice about the baseline?

2 What do you notice about the baseline variability?

3 What type of decelerations, if any, are present?

4 What do you notice about the uterine activity?

5 What is the most probable cause of fetal heart rate abnormality shown on this trace?

6 What treatment and/or intervention would you consider necessary for this fetal heart rate pattern?

NOTES

1

2

3

4

5

6

ANALYSIS

1 Baseline – difficult to ascertain whether true baseline or prolonged deceleration as no previous CTG

2 Variability little or absent

3 Prolonged deceleration – see baseline comment

4 No contractions monitored

5 Rapid progress in labour
  Possible cord compression

6 Change maternal position
  Give facial oxygen
  Exclude cord prolapse
  Prepare for delivery

OUTCOME

15.40 hours
Second stage of labour confirmed

15.50 hours
Straight forceps delivery
Live boy
Apgar score 3/1 9/5
Birthweight 3.200 kg
Cord around neck × 1

HISTORY

37-year-old gravida I, para 0

Past history
Nil relevant

Antenatal period
Amniocentesis performed at 17 weeks –
indication, maternal age; result shows normal
karyotype
Admitted at 26 weeks with polyhydramnios

31 weeks
Ultrasound scan shows fetal ascites

33 weeks
Contracting 1 in 5 minutes for 2 hours

Labour

20.00 hours
Abdominal decompression performed – 6
litres of amniotic fluid drained

20.50 hours
Cervical os 4 cm dilated
CTG reactive, baseline 120 b.p.m.
External monitoring

22.00 hours
Cervical os 5 cm dilated

22.15 hours
CTG

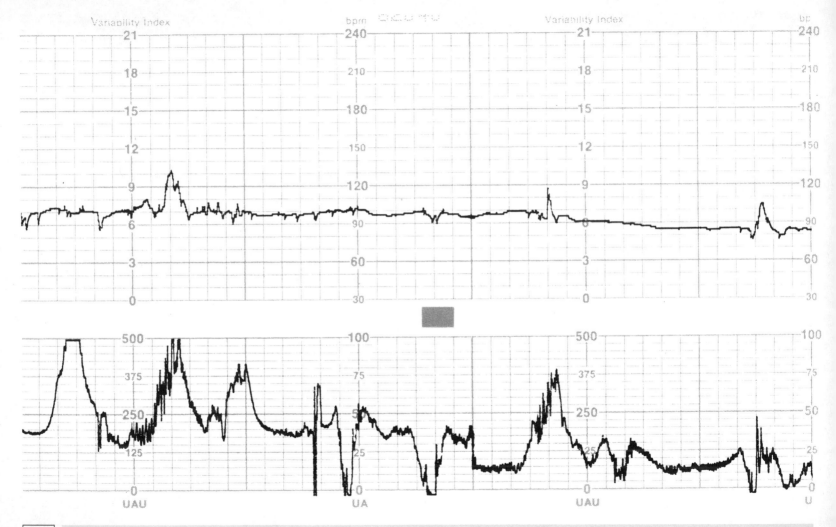

CTG

1 What do you notice about the baseline?

2 What do you notice about the baseline variability?

3 What type of decelerations, if any, are present?

4 What do you notice about the uterine activity?

5 What is the most probable cause of fetal heart rate abnormality shown on this trace?

6 What treatment and/or intervention would you consider necessary for this fetal heart rate pattern?

NOTES

1

2

3

4

5

6

ANALYSIS

1 Baseline 90–100 b.p.m. on portion of CTG

2 Variability – external recording, therefore
  not accurate; appears to be little or absent

3 No decelerations, occasional acceleration

4 Contractions not monitored adequately

5 Falling baseline, previously 120 b.p.m.
  In view of abdominal decompression and
  amount of liquor removed, placental
  abruption must be considered
  Cord occlusion possible
  Fetal hypoxia suggested although
  accelerations a reassuring sign

6 Vaginal examination to exclude cord
  prolapse and assess cervical dilation
  Change maternal position
  Give facial oxygen
  Decision to deliver will be difficult in view of
  diagnosis of fetal ascites of unknown origin

OUTCOME

22.50 hours
Second stage of labour diagnosed

23.10 hours
Rotational forceps delivery
Live boy
Apgar score 1/1 3/5
Birthweight 2.320 kg
Baby – hydropic
Neonatal death at 12 hours old
200 ml retroplacental clot

HISTORY

20-year-old gravida I, para 0

Past history
Nil relevant

Antenatal period
Breech presentation confirmed on ultrasound scan at 38 weeks
Admitted in labour at 39 weeks, contracting 1 in 5 minutes

Labour

23.30 hours
Cervical os 4 cm dilated
Artificial rupture of membranes – clear liquor draining
Fetal scalp electrode applied
Intrauterine pressure catheter inserted

00.57 hours
Epidural analgesia commenced

02.00 hours
Cervical os 7 cm dilated
CTG reactive
Baseline 150 b.p.m.

03.00 hours
Meconium-stained liquor noted
Maternal temperature 36°C

03.50 hours
Cervical os 9.5 cm dilated
CTG

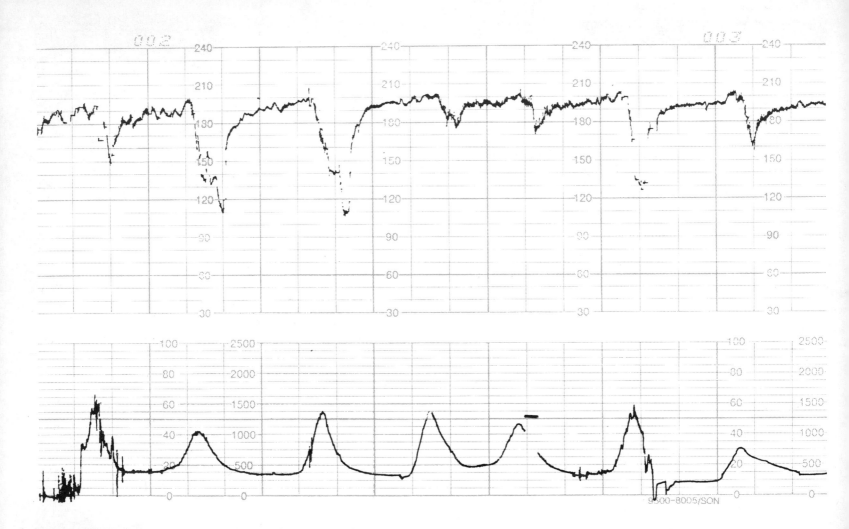

CTG

1 What do you notice about the baseline?

2 What do you notice about the baseline variability?

3 What type of decelerations, if any, are present?

4 What do you notice about the uterine activity?

5 What is the most probable cause of fetal heart rate abnormality shown on this trace?

6 What treatment and/or intervention would you consider necessary for this fetal heart rate pattern?

NOTES

1

2

3

4

5

6

ANALYSIS

1 Baseline 190–200 b.p.m.

2 Variability 5 b.p.m.

3 Variable decelerations

4 Contracting 4 in 10 minutes

5 Maternal temperature normal. Baseline increasing, variability diminishing, variable decelerations – fetal hypoxia should be considered

6 Prepare for delivery
  Change maternal position
  Give facial oxygen
  Increase intravenous fluids

OUTCOME

04.30 hours
Caesarean section performed
Live boy
Apgar score 6/1 9/5
Birthweight 3.430 kg

HISTORY

16-year-old gravida I, para 0

Past history
Nil relevant

Antenatal period
Normal
Admitted at 41 weeks with contractions for 5 hours

Labour

17.05 hours
Cervical os 4 cm dilated
Artificial rupture of membranes – clear liquor draining
Fetal scalp electrode applied
Intrauterine pressure catheter inserted

17.15 hours
Pethidine 100 mg and Sparine 25 mg given intramuscularly

19.15 hours
Cervical os 4 cm dilated
Syntocinon infusion commenced

22.00 hours
Cervical os 4 cm dilated

24.00 hours
Cervical os 4 cm dilated
Clear liquor
Syntocinon infusing at 8 mU/min
Maternal temperature 36.4°C

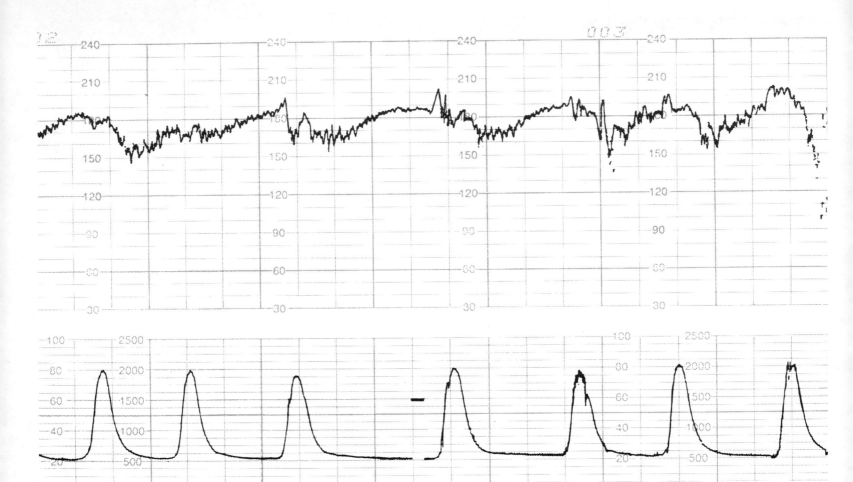

CTG

1 What do you notice about the baseline?

2 What do you notice about the baseline variability?

3 What type of decelerations, if any, are present?

4 What do you notice about the uterine activity?

5 What is the most probable cause of fetal heart rate abnormality shown on this trace?

6 What treatment and/or intervention would you consider necessary for this fetal heart rate pattern?

NOTES

1

2

3

4

5

6

ANALYSIS

1 Baseline 180–190 b.p.m.

2 Variability 5–10 b.p.m.

3 Late decelerations

4 Contracting 3–4 in 10 minutes

5 Fetal tachycardia, maternal temperature
normal, late decelerations – fetal hypoxia
despite variability being within normal limits

6 Change maternal position
Give facial oxygen
Increase intravenous infusion
Stop Syntocinon infusion
Fetal blood sampling is indicated
Prepare for delivery, particularly in view of
failure to progress

OUTCOME

02.00 hours
Cervix 6 cm dilated
Fetal blood sampling performed: pH 7.23,
base excess –6
CTG continues as before, late decelerations
becoming more severe

03.00 hours
Caesarean section performed
Live girl
Apgar score 7/1 10/5
Birthweight 3.240 kg

CASE STUDY

47

HISTORY

18-year-old gravida I, para 0

Past history
Nil relevant

Antenatal period
Normal
Admitted at 36 weeks with history of heavy, fresh bleeding per vagina for 2 hours – sudden onset; complaining of abdominal pain
On examination: abdomen tense and tender; moderate amount fresh bleeding per vagina
Admission CTG

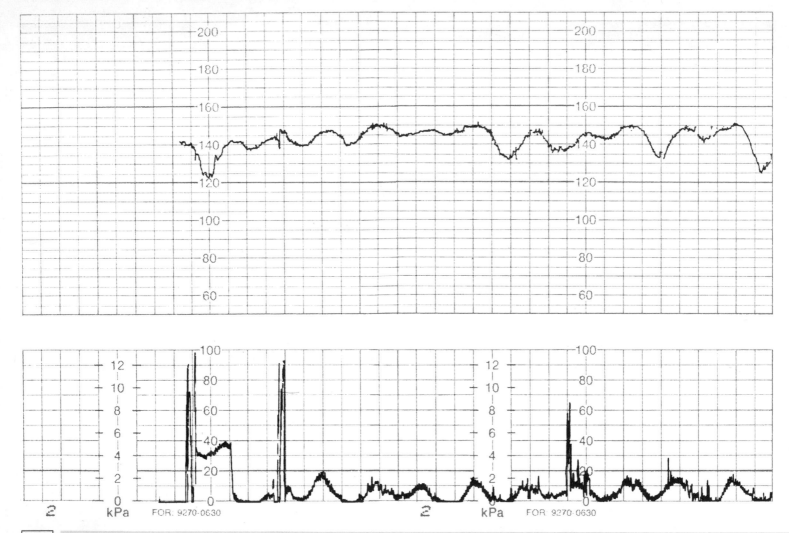

FOR. 9270-0630

FOR. 9270-0630

CTG

1 What do you notice about the baseline?

2 What do you notice about the baseline variability?

3 What type of decelerations, if any, are present?

4 What do you notice about the uterine activity?

5 What is the most probable cause of fetal heart rate abnormality shown on this trace?

6 What treatment and/or intervention would you consider necessary for this fetal heart rate pattern?

NOTES

1

2

3

4

5

6

ANALYSIS

1 Baseline 145–150 b.p.m.

2 Variability – external recording, therefore not accurate; appears to be little or absent

3 Late decelerations

4 Uterine irritability

5 Reduced placental blood flow due to placental abruption – fetal hypoxia

6 Prepare for delivery
  Change maternal position
  Give facial oxygen

OUTCOME

Ultrasound scan performed – posterior upper segment of placenta
Cervix 1 cm long, cervical os 2 cm dilated
Caesarean section performed
Baby girl
Apgar score 0/1 7/5 9/10
Resuscitated successfully
Birthweight 2.690 kg
Couvelaire uterus noted
Baby discharged at 3 weeks

HISTORY

36-year-old gravida III, para II

Past history
Nil relevant

Antenatal period
Admitted at 33 weeks with raised blood
pressure
Diminished fetal movements
Ultrasound scan shows asymmetrical growth
retardation and reduced liquor volume
Admission CTG

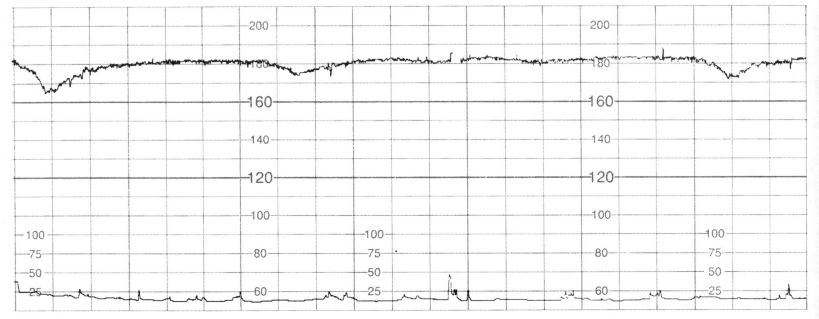

CTG

1 What do you notice about the baseline?

2 What do you notice about the baseline variability?

3 What type of decelerations, if any, are present?

4 What do you notice about the uterine activity?

5 What is the most probable cause of fetal heart rate abnormality shown on this trace?

6 What treatment and/or intervention would you consider necessary for this fetal heart rate pattern?

NOTES

1

2

3

4

5

6

ANALYSIS

1 Baseline 180 b.p.m.

2 Variability – external recording, therefore not accurate; appears to be virtually absent

3 Shallow decelerations, cannot be classified in absence of contractions

4 No contractions

5 History of intrauterine growth retardation, diminished liquor volume, diminished fetal movements, fetal tachycardia, decreased variability, decelerations occurring without contractions – fetal hypoxia

6 Give facial oxygen
Change maternal position
Prepare for delivery

OUTCOME

Emergency caesarean section performed
Live boy
Apgar score 1/1 4/5
Birthweight 1.470 kg
True knot in cord
Baby transferred to neonatal unit
Discharged at 4 weeks

49

PART 1

HISTORY

27-year-old gravida II, para I

Past history
Nil relevant

Antenatal period
Normal
Admitted at 43 weeks for routine CTG

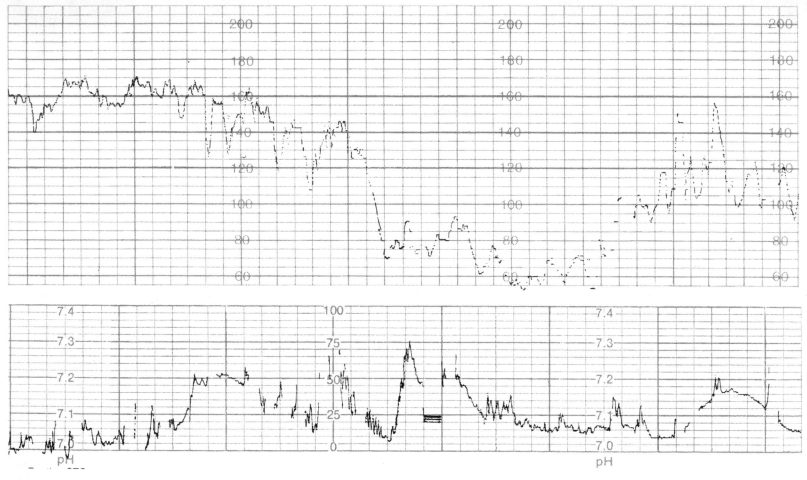

Routine CTG.

CTG

1 What do you notice about the baseline?

2 What do you notice about the baseline variability?

3 What type of decelerations, if any, are present?

4 What do you notice about the uterine activity?

5 What is the most probable cause of fetal heart rate abnormality shown on this trace?

6 What treatment and/or intervention would you consider necessary for this fetal heart rate pattern?

NOTES

1

2

3

4

5

6

ANALYSIS

1 Baseline 150–160 b.p.m.

2 Variability external recording, therefore not
  accurate; appears within normal limits

3 Prolonged deceleration

4 Occasional tightening, no contractions

5 Cord occlusion is a possibility
  Note gestation; placental insufficiency
  resulting in fetal hypoxia must be
  considered

6 Prepare for delivery
  Change maternal position
  Give facial oxygen
  Vaginal examination to assess cervix
  If deceleration recovers and cervix
  favourable, consider surgical induction of
  labour

OUTCOME

15.00 hours
Surgical induction of labour performed
Cervix 1.5 cm long, cervical os 3 cm dilated
Artificial rupture of membranes – fresh
meconium-stained liquor draining
Fetal scalp electrode applied
Contractions monitored externally
Contracting spontaneously

15.45 hours
Pethidine 100 mg and Sparine 25 mg given
intramuscularly

16.00 hours
CTG – see Part 2, page 266.

49

PART 2

OUTCOME [CONTINUED]

16.00 hours
CTG

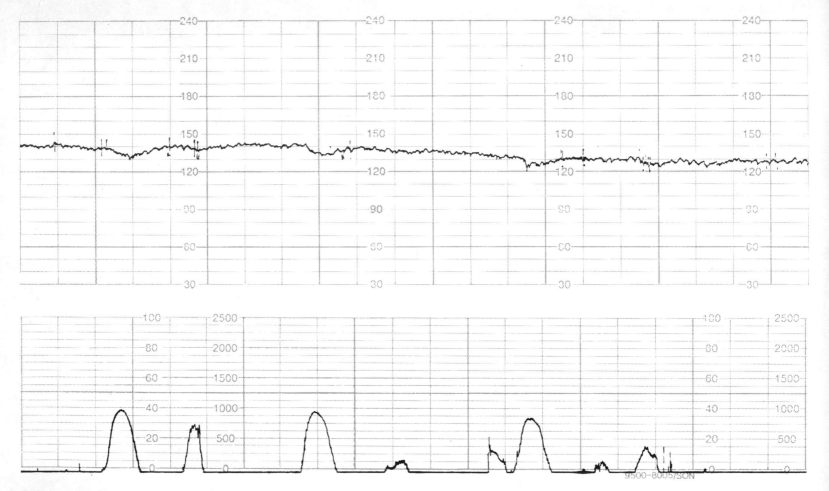

CTG at 16.00 hours.

CTG	NOTES
1 What do you notice about the baseline?	1
2 What do you notice about the baseline variability?	2
3 What type of decelerations, if any, are present?	3
4 What do you notice about the uterine activity?	4
5 What is the most probable cause of fetal heart rate abnormality shown on this trace?	5
6 What treatment and/or intervention would you consider necessary for this fetal heart rate pattern?	6

ANALYSIS

1 Baseline 140–150 b.p.m.

2 Less than 5 b.p.m.

3 Possibly very shallow late decelerations

4 Contracting irregularly, varying in strength; inadequately monitored

5 Pethidine given 15 minutes prior to portion of CTG; however, in view of previous CTG and fresh meconium-stained liquor, fetal hypoxia must be considered

6 Change maternal position
  Give facial oxygen
  Commence intravenous fluids
  Fetal blood sampling is indicated
  If pattern persists, prepare for delivery

OUTCOME

17.00 hours
Cervical os 5 cm dilated
Fetal blood sampling performed: pH 7.20, base excess −10
Caesarean section performed
Live girl
Apgar score 9/1 9/5
Birthweight 4.560 kg
Cord around neck ×1 and around leg × 2

CASE STUDY

50

PART 1

HISTORY

23-year-old gravida I, para 0

Past history
Nil relevant

Antenatal period
Normal
Admitted at 39 weeks with spontaneous
rupture of membranes – meconium-stained
liquor draining

Labour

15.00 hours
Cervix 0.5 cm long, cervical os 1 cm dilated
Fetal scalp electrode applied
Intrauterine pressure catheter inserted
Labour augmented with Syntocinon
CTG: normal, baseline 145 b.p.m., reactive

19.00 hours
Cervical os 3 cm dilated
Occasional variable deceleration noted, CTG
otherwise normal

03.00 hours
Cervical os 6 cm dilated
Maternal temperature 38.2°C
Fetal tachycardia – 170 b.p.m.
Variability normal
Syntocinon infusing at 12 mU/min

06.00 hours
Cervical os 9 cm dilated
CTG

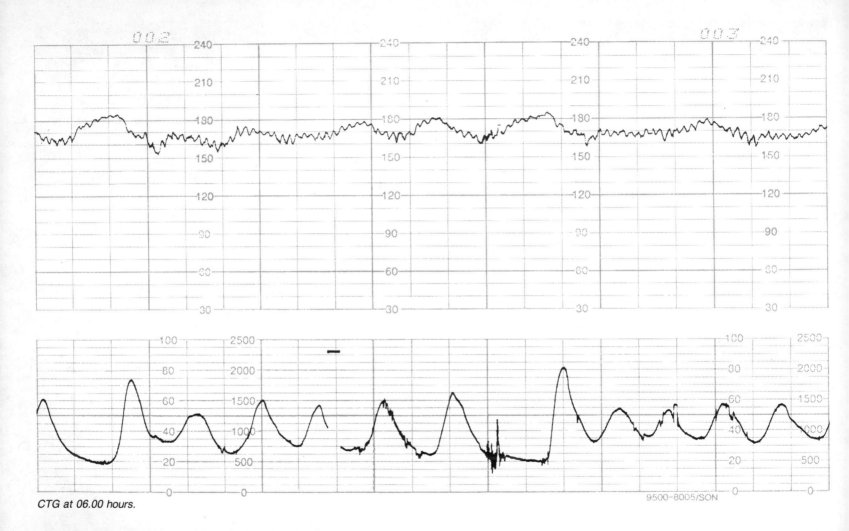

CTG at 06.00 hours.

CTG	NOTES
1 What do you notice about the baseline?	1
2 What do you notice about the baseline variability?	
3 What type of decelerations, if any, are present?	2
4 What do you notice about the uterine activity?	3
5 What is the most probable cause of fetal heart rate abnormality shown on this trace?	4
6 What treatment and/or intervention would you consider necessary for this fetal heart rate pattern?	5
	6

ANALYSIS

1 Baseline 170–180 b.p.m.

2 Variability virtually absent; sinusoidal pattern

3 Late decelerations

4 Contracting 6 in 10 minutes, high uterine resting tone

5 In view of fetal tachycardia and late decelerations, sinusoidal pattern not idiopathic – fetal hypoxia

6 Change maternal position
Give facial oxygen
Increase intravenous infusion
Stop Syntocinon infusion
Fetal blood sampling contraindicated in view of maternal pyrexia
Prepare for delivery

OUTCOME

Second stage of labour diagnosed
Syntocinon infusing at 6 mU/min

08.00 hours
CTG – see Part 2, page 274.

OUTCOME [CONTINUED]

08.00 hours
CTG

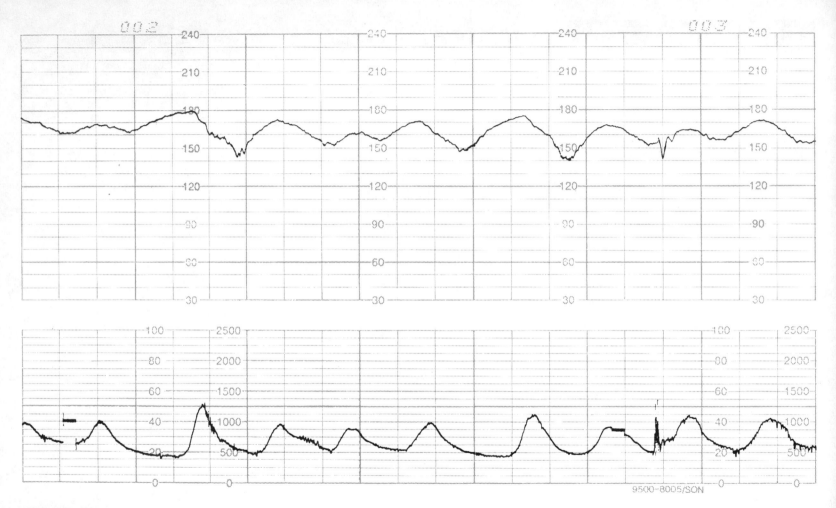

CTG at 08.00 hours.

CTG

1 What do you notice about the baseline?

2 What do you notice about the baseline variability?

3 What type of decelerations, if any, are present?

4 What do you notice about the uterine activity?

5 What is the most probable cause of fetal heart rate abnormality shown on this trace?

6 What treatment and/or intervention would you consider necessary for this fetal heart rate pattern?

NOTES

1

2

3

4

5

6

ANALYSIS

1 Baseline 170–180 b.p.m.

2 Variability absent

3 Late decelerations

4 Contracting 4 in 10 minutes

5 Fetal hypoxia

6 Change maternal position
  Give facial oxygen
  Stop Syntocinon infusion
  Increase intravenous infusion
  Prepare for delivery

OUTCOME

09.15 hours
Failure to progress in second stage of labour
Caesarean section performed
Stillborn girl
Birthweight 3.480 kg

Prolonged

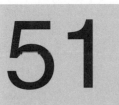
HISTORY

33-year-old gravida II, para I

Past history
Nil relevant

Antenatal period
Normal
Admitted at 36 weeks with abdominal pain, fresh bleeding per vagina and contracting 1 in 3 minutes
Speculum examination performed – 30 ml of fresh blood in vagina
Ultrasound scan performed – upper segment placenta

Labour

04.30 hours
Cervical os 3 cm dilated
Artificial rupture of membranes – heavily blood-stained liquor
Fetal scalp electrode applied
Intrauterine pressure catheter inserted

04.55 hours
CTG

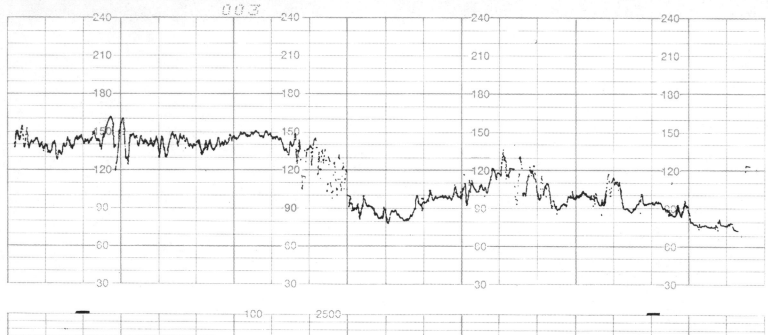

9500-8005/SON

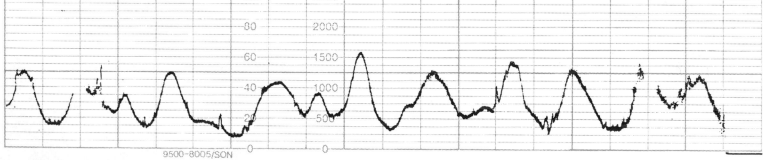

CTG	NOTES
1 What do you notice about the baseline?	1
2 What do you notice about the baseline variability?	
3 What type of decelerations, if any, are present?	2
4 What do you notice about the uterine activity?	3
5 What is the most probable cause of fetal heart rate abnormality shown on this trace?	4
6 What treatment and/or intervention would you consider necessary for this fetal heart rate pattern?	
	5
	6

LIVERPOOL
JOHN MOORES UNIVERSITY
AVRIL ROBARTS LRC
TEL. 0151 231 4022

ANALYSIS

1 Baseline 135–145 b.p.m.

2 Variability 5–15 b.p.m.

3 Prolonged deceleration

4 Contracting 5 in 10 minutes, varying in strength

5 Possible further placental abruption resulting in diminished oxygen transfer to the fetus, causing fetal hypoxia

6 Vaginal examination to assess cervical dilation
Change maternal position
Give facial oxygen
Prepare for delivery

OUTCOME

05.25 hours
Caesarean section performed
Live boy
Apgar score 3/1 10/5
Birthweight 2.610 kg
300 ml retroplacental clot

HISTORY

23-year-old gravida II, para 0 + 1

Past history
Nil relevant

Antenatal period
Normal
Admitted at 41 weeks with spontaneous rupture of membranes – slightly meconium-stained liquor draining

Labour

21.40 hours
Cervical os 4 cm dilated
Fetal scalp electrode applied
Contractions monitored externally

22.20 hours
Epidural analgesia commenced

23.15 hours
Cervical os 6 cm dilated

23.30 hours
Epidural top-up given

24.00 hours
Occasional variable decelerations noted

00.50 hours
CTG

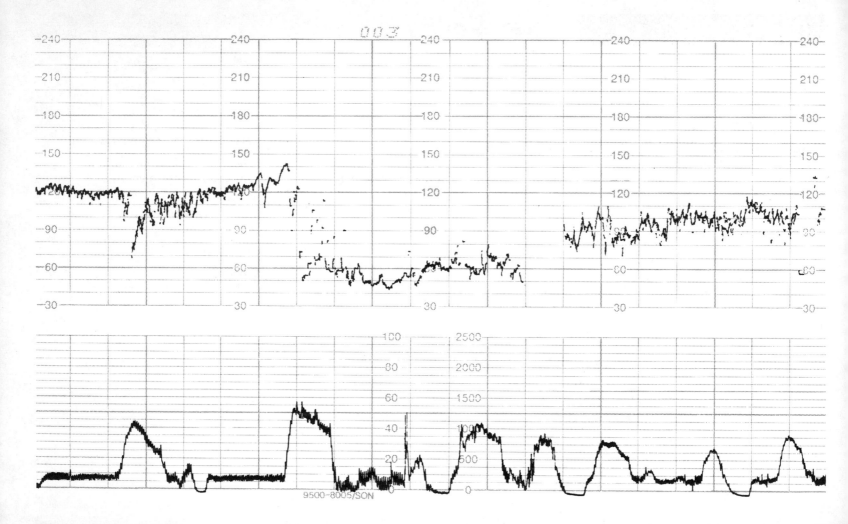

003

9500-8005/SON

CTG

1 What do you notice about the baseline?

2 What do you notice about the baseline variability?

3 What type of decelerations, if any, are present?

4 What do you notice about the uterine activity?

5 What is the most probable cause of fetal heart rate abnormality shown on this trace?

6 What treatment and/or intervention would you consider necessary for this fetal heart rate pattern?

NOTES

1

2

3

4

5

6

ANALYSIS

1 Baseline 120 b.p.m.

2 Variability 5 b.p.m.

3 Prolonged decelerations

4 Contracting 4–5 in 10 minutes, varying in strength

5 Previous variable decelerations – cord occlusion probable, resulting in fetal hypoxia

6 Vaginal examination to assess cervical dilation and to exclude cord prolapse
Change maternal position
Give facial oxygen
Fetal blood sampling when deceleration recovers
If no recovery, deliver

OUTCOME

Cervical os 8 cm dilated
No cord prolapse
Fetal blood sampling attempted – failed
Fetal heart returned to baseline 120–130 b.p.m., with occasional variable decelerations

03.33 hours
Second stage of labour diagnosed

04.15 hours
Spontaneous vertex delivery
Live boy
Apgar score 1/1 7/5
Birthweight 3.140 kg
True knot in cord

HISTORY

21-year-old gravida I, para 0

Past history
Ovarian cystectomy 3 years ago

Antenatal period
Normal
Admitted at 39 weeks, contracting 1 in 5
minutes for 3 hours

Labour

11.30 hours
Cervical os 2 cm dilated
Artificial rupture of membranes – clear liquor
draining
Fetal scalp electrode applied
Intrauterine pressure catheter inserted

14.30 hours
Cervical os 4 cm dilated
Epidural analgesia commenced

15.30 hours
Epidural top-up given

16.15 hours
CTG

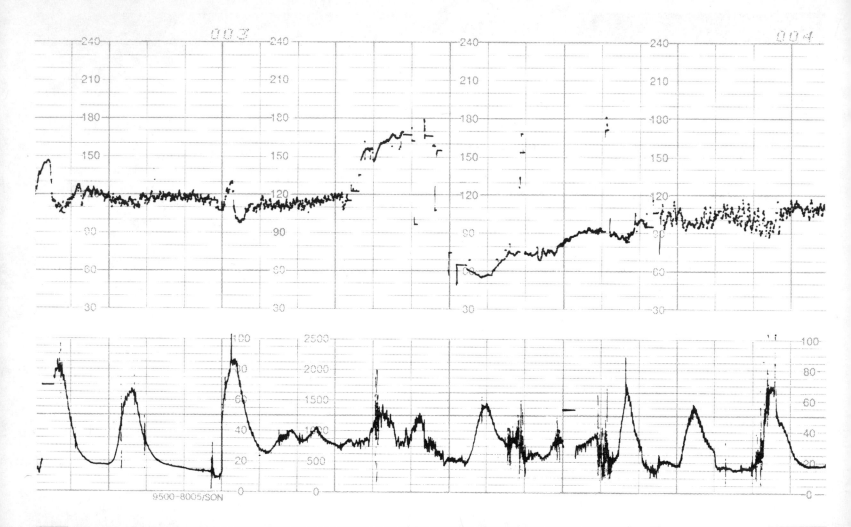

9500-8005/SON

CTG

1 What do you notice about the baseline?

2 What do you notice about the baseline variability?

3 What type of decelerations, if any, are present?

4 What do you notice about the uterine activity?

5 What is the most probable cause of fetal heart rate abnormality shown on this trace?

6 What treatment and/or intervention would you consider necessary for this fetal heart rate pattern?

NOTES

1

2

3

4

5

6

ANALYSIS

1 Baseline 110–120 b.p.m.

2 Variability 5–10 b.p.m.

3 Prolonged decelerations

4 Contracting 4–5 in 10 minutes, varying in strength

5 Deceleration occurs immediately after vaginal examination

6 Change maternal position
  Give facial oxygen
  Increase intravenous fluids
  Consider fetal blood sampling when fetal heart rate returns to normal
  If no recovery, prepare for delivery
  Observe for further abnormalities

OUTCOME

CTG returns to normal – no further decelerations

18.15 hours
Second stage of labour diagnosed

19.40 hours
Straight forceps delivery
Live girl
Apgar score 9/1 9/5
Birthweight 3.480 kg
No cord around neck

PART 4

Summary chart: risk assessment

Risk assessment chart

To minimise the risk of untoward occurrences/outcomes, the checklist in Table 1 has been compiled in relation to cardiotocography and should be used in conjunction with your employer's policies, protocols or guidelines and any rules, codes of practice and guidelines concerning the framework within which you practise as a doctor or midwife. For midwives, these will be those set out by the United Kingdom Central Council (UKCC) for Nursing, Midwifery and Health Visiting. For doctors they will be those of the employer.

Both groups must be familiar with any guidelines and/or protocols relevant to their practice set out by an NHS trust or other place of work outside the NHS.

Table 1 Checklist of questions

	Yes	No
Are you confident and competent in the interpretation of the CTG?	☐	☐
Have you been trained and are you familiar with all the fetal monitoring equipment used in the clinical setting in which you work?	☐	☐
Are you aware of the facilities and personnel available for the repair and maintenance of equipment?	☐	☐
Are you satisfied with your knowledge of the research evidence, with regard to fetal monitoring, and do you base your practice upon this?	☐	☐
Are you comfortable in communicating any concerns regarding the interpretation of a CTG?	☐	☐
Do you obtain consent (informed) from women prior to commencing continuous fetal monitoring?	☐	☐
Do you attend regular multidisciplinary updating and training events in the interpretation of CTGs?	☐	☐
Is your record-keeping maintained to the highest standard; is it clear, concise, legible and unambiguous?	☐	☐
When making records relating to a CTG, in the case notes, do you describe the baseline, variability, reactivity and presence or absence of any decelerations as opposed to writing 'normal' or 'satisfactory'?	☐	☐
Is there a means of storing CTGs within the case notes that ensures that they do not get lost or damaged?	☐	☐

If the answer to any of the questions in Table 1 is 'No', then ask yourself 'What must I do about it?' Is it a matter for you, your colleagues, your supervisor of midwives, your manager?

The UKCC distributes the documents specified in Table 2 to all practitioners on the register. They are revised from time to time and it is the responsibility of each midwife to be familiar with their contents and refer to them as and when appropriate. If you do not have copies of any of the UKCC documents on the list, then write to the UKCC at: 23 Portland Place, London W1N 4JT

Table 2 Checklist of documents relating to practice

	Yes	No
Do you have a copy of the most up-to-date UKCC rules, codes and guidelines for professional practice and are you familiar with them?	☐	☐
Midwives' rules and code of practice 1998	☐	☐
Code of Professional Conduct 1992	☐	☐
Scope of Professional Practice 1992	☐	☐
Guidelines for Professional Practice 1996	☐	☐
Guidelines for records and record keeping 1998	☐	☐
Are there trust documents relating to any of your practice and are you familiar with them?	☐	☐
NHS trust/non-NHS guidelines/protocols available	☐	☐

INDEX

Numbers in bold refer to CTG examples